Innovative Approaches to Addressing Pediatric Mental Health

Editors

ROBERT T. AMMERMAN
CRAIG A. ERICKSON

PEDIATRIC CLINICS OF NORTH AMERICA

www.pediatric.theclinics.com

Consulting Editor
TINA L. CHENG

December 2024 • Volume 71 • Number 6

ELSEVIER

1600 John F. Kennedy Boulevard • Suite 1800 • Philadelphia, Pennsylvania, 19103-2899

http://www.theclinics.com

THE PEDIATRIC CLINICS OF NORTH AMERICA Volume 71, Number 6
December 2024 ISSN 0031-3955, ISBN-13: 978-0-443-29362-7

Editor: Kerry Holland
Developmental Editor: Anirban Mukherjee

The Pediatric Clinics of North America (ISSN 0031-3955) is published bimonthly by Elsevier Inc., 360 Park Avenue South, New York, NY 10010-1710. Months of issue are February, April, June, August, October, and December. Periodicals postage paid at New York, NY and additional mailing offices. Subscription prices are $290.00 per year (US individuals), $368.00 per year (Canadian individuals), $440.00 per year (international individuals), $100.00 per year (US students and residents), $100.00 per year (Canadian students and residents), and $165.00 per year (international residents and students). For institutional access pricing please contact Customer Service via the contact information below. To receive students/resident rare, orders must be accompanied by name of affiliated institution, date of term, and the signature of program/residency coordinator on institution letterhead. Orders will be billed at individual rate until proof of status is received. Foreign air speed delivery is included in all *Clinics* subscription prices. All prices are subject to change without notice. Orders, claims, and journal inquiries: Please visit our Support Hub page https://service.elsevier.com for assistance.

Reprints. For copies of 100 or more, of articles in this publication, please contact the Commercial Reprints Department, Elsevier Inc., 360 Park Avenue South, New York, NY 10010-1710. Tel.: 212-633-3874; Fax: 212-633-3820; E-mail: reprints@elsevier.com.

The Pediatric Clinics of North America is also published in Spanish by McGraw-Hill Inter-americana Editores S.A., Mexico City, Mexico; in Portuguese by Riechmann and Affonso Editores, Rua Comandante Coelho 1085, CEP 21250, Rio de Janeiro, Brazil; and in Greek by Althayia SA, Athens, Greece.

The Pediatric Clinics of North America is covered in *MEDLINE/PubMed (Index Medicus), Excerpta Medica, Current Contents, Current Contents/Clinical Medicine, Science Citation Index, ASCA, ISI/BIOMED*, and *BIOSIS*.

Printed in the United States of America.

JOURNAL TITLE: Pediatric Clinics of North America
ISSUE: 71.6

PROGRAM OBJECTIVE

The goal of the *Pediatric Clinics of North America* is to keep practicing physicians and residents up to date with current clinical practice in pediatrics by providing timely articles reviewing the state-of-the-art in patient care.

TARGET AUDIENCE

All practicing pediatricians, physicians, and healthcare professionals who provide patient care to pediatric patients.

LEARNING OBJECTIVES

Upon completion of this activity, participants will be able to:

1. Review the various mental health screenings and measurements in children and adolescents.
2. Discuss how pediatric clinicians can maximize the effectiveness of interventions that address mental health concerns.
3. Recognize the COVID-19 pandemic has exacerbated mental health concerns among children and adolescents.

ACCREDITATIONS

Physician Credit

The Elsevier Office of Continuing Medical Education (EOCME) is accredited by the Accreditation Council for Continuing Medical Education (ACCME) to provide continuing medical education for physicians.

The EOCME designates this journal-based activity for a maximum of 12 *AMA PRA Category 1 Credit(s)*™

Physicians should claim only the credit commensurate with the extent of their participation in the activity.

All other healthcare professionals requesting continuing education credit for this journal-based activity will be issued a certificate of participation.

ABP Maintenance of Certification Credit

Successful completion of this CME activity, which includes participation in the activity and individual assessment of and feedback to the learner, enables the learner to earn up to 12 MOC points in the American Board of Pediatrics' (ABP) Maintenance of Certification (MOC) program. It is the CME activity provider's responsibility to submit learner completion information to ACCME for the purpose of granting ABP MOC credit.

DISCLOSURE OF RELEVANT FINANCIAL RELATIONSHIPS

The EOCME assesses conflict of interest with its instructors, faculty, planners, and other individuals who are in a position to control the content of CME activities. All relevant conflicts of interest that are identified are thoroughly vetted by EOCME for fair balance, scientific objectivity, and patient care recommendations. EOCME is committed to providing its learners with CME activities that promote improvements or quality in healthcare and not a specific proprietary business or a commercial interest.

The authors and editors listed below have identified no financial relationships or relationships to products or devices they have with ineligible companies related to the content of this CME activity:
Craig A. Erickson, MD; Robert T. Ammerman, PhD; Ann H. Farrell, PhD; Peter Szatmari, MD, FRCPC, FRSC; Tracy Vaillancourt, PhD, FRSC; Marie Reilly, MD; Carol Weitzman, MD; David W. Willis, MD, FAAP; Dayna Long, MD; Kay Johnson, MPH, EdM; Rachel B. Herbst, PhD; Alexandra M.S. Corley, MD, MPH; Emily McTate, PhD; Julie M. Gettings, PhD; Chuan Mei Lee, MD, MA: Jayme Congdon, MD, MSc; Christina Joy, MD; Barry Sarvet, MD; Jessica M. McClure, PsyD; Melissa A. Young, PsyD; Yu Chen, PhD; Danruo Zhong, PhD; Erin Roby, PhD; Caitlin Canfield, PhD; Alan Mendelsohn, MD; Heather Forkey, MD; Jessica Griffin, PsyD; Donna A. Ruch, PhD; Jennifer L. Hughes, PhD, MPH; Jeffrey A. Bridge, PhD; Cynthia A. Fontanella, PhD; Chidiogo Anyigbo, MD, MPH; Sarah J. Beal, PhD; Joyce Y. Lee, PhD; Laura M. Gottlieb, MD, MPH; Gary Maslow, MD, MPH; Richard Chung, MD; Nicole Heilbron, PhD; Barbara Keith Walter, PhD, MPH; Lawrence S. Wissow, MD, MPH; Laura P. Richardson, MD, MPH

The planning committee and staff listed below have identified no financial relationships or relationships to products or devices they have with ineligible companies related to the content of this CME activity:
Kerry Holland; Shyamala Kavikumaran; Michelle Littlejohn; Patrick J. Manley; Anirban Mukherjee

UNAPPROVED/OFF-LABEL USE DISCLOSURE

The EOCME requires CME faculty to disclose to the participants:

1. When products or procedures being discussed are off-label, unlabelled, experimental, and/or investigational (not US Food and Drug Administration [FDA] approved); and
2. Any limitations on the information presented, such as data that are preliminary or that represent ongoing research, interim analyses, and/or unsupported opinions. Faculty may discuss information about pharmaceutical agents that is outside of FDA-approved labelling. This information is intended solely for CME and is not intended to promote off-label use of these medications. If you have any questions, contact the medical affairs department of the manufacturer for the most recent prescribing information.

TO ENROLL

To enroll in the *Pediatric Clinics of North America* Continuing Medical Education program, call customer service at 1-800-654-2452 or sign up online at http://www.theclinics.com/home/cme. The CME program is available to subscribers for an additional annual fee of USD 313.00.

METHOD OF PARTICIPATION

In order to claim credit, participants must complete the following:

1. Complete enrolment as indicated above.
2. Read the activity.
3. Complete the CME Test and Evaluation. Participants must achieve a score of 70% on the test. All CME Tests and Evaluations must be completed online.

CME INQUIRIES/SPECIAL NEEDS

For all CME inquiries or special needs, please contact elsevierCME@elsevier.com.

Contributors

CONSULTING EDITOR

TINA L. CHENG, MD, MPH
BK Rachford Professor and Chair of Pediatrics, University of Cincinnati, Director, Cincinnati Children's Research Foundation, Chief Medical Officer, Cincinnati Children's Hospital Medical Center, Cincinnati, Ohio, USA

EDITORS

ROBERT T. AMMERMAN, PhD
Professor of Pediatrics, Cincinnati Children's Hospital Medical Center, University of Cincinnati College of Medicine, Cincinnati, Ohio, USA

CRAIG A. ERICKSON, MD
Research Director and Research Endowed Professor, Cincinnati Children's Hospital Medical Center, University of Cincinnati College of Medicine, Cincinnati, Ohio, USA

AUTHORS

CHIDIOGO ANYIGBO, MD, MPH
Assistant Professor, Division of General and Community Pediatrics, Cincinnati Children's Hospital Medical Center, Department of Pediatrics, University of Cincinnati College of Medicine, Cincinnati, Ohio, USA

SARAH J. BEAL, PhD
Professor, Divisions of Behavioral Medicine and Clinical Psychology and General and Community Pediatrics, Cincinnati Children's Hospital Medical Center, Department of Pediatrics, University of Cincinnati College of Medicine, Cincinnati, Ohio, USA

JEFFREY A. BRIDGE, PhD
Epidemiologist and Director, Center for Suicide Prevention and Research, The Abigail Wexner Research Institute, Nationwide Children's Hospital, Professor of Pediatrics, Psychiatry and Behavioral Health, Department of Pediatrics, The Ohio State University College of Medicine, Epidemiologist and Director, Big Lots Behavioral Health Services, Division of Child and Family Psychiatry, Nationwide Children's Hospital, Nationwide Foundation Endowed Chair of Innovation and Professor, Department of Psychiatry and Behavioral Health, The Ohio State University College of Medicine, Columbus, Ohio, USA

CAITLIN CANFIELD, PhD
Assistant Professor, Division of Developmental-Behavioral Pediatrics, Department of Pediatrics, NYU Grossman School of Medicine, New York, New York, USA

YU CHEN, PhD
Postdoctoral Fellow, Division of Developmental-Behavioral Pediatrics, Department of Pediatrics, NYU Grossman School of Medicine, New York, New York, USA

RICHARD CHUNG, MD
Distinguished Endowed Chair, Department of Pediatrics, Perelmen School of Medicine, University of Pennsylvania, Attending Physician, Division of Adolescent Medicine, Senior Medical Director for Enterprise Adolescent Medicine, Population Health Management, and Transitions, Children's Hospital of Philadelphia, Philadelphia, Pennsylvania, USA

JAYME CONGDON, MD, MS
Assistant Professor, Department of Pediatrics, Philip R. Lee Institute for Health Policy Studies, University of California, San Francisco, San Francisco, California, USA

ALEXANDRA M.S. CORLEY, MD, MPH
Assistant Professor, University of Cincinnati College of Medicine, General Pediatrician, Division of General and Community Pediatrics, Cincinnati Children's Hospital Medical Center, Cincinnati, Ohio, USA

ANN H. FARRELL, PhD
Assistant Professor, Department of Child and Youth Studies, Brock University, St Catharines, Ontario, Canada

CYNTHIA A. FONTANELLA, PhD
Principal Investigator, Center for Suicide Prevention and Research, The Abigail Wexner Research Institute, Nationwide Children's Hospital, Professor, Department of Psychiatry and Behavioral Health, The Ohio State University College of Medicine, Columbus, Ohio, USA

HEATHER FORKEY, MD
Professor, Department of Pediatrics, UMass Chan Medical School, UMass Memorial Children's Medical Center, Worcester, Massachusetts, USA

JULIE M. GETTINGS, PhD
Assistant Professor, Department of Clinical Psychiatry, Perelman School of Medicine, University of Pennsylvania, Pediatric Psychologist, Department of Child and Adolescent Psychiatry and Behavioral Sciences, Children's Hospital of Philadelphia, Philadelphia, Pennsylvania, USA

LAURA M. GOTTLIEB, MD, MPH
Professor, Department of Family and Community Medicine, School of Medicine, University of California San Francisco, Director, Social Interventions Research and Evaluation Network, University of California, San Francisco, San Francisco, California, USA

JESSICA GRIFFIN, PsyD
Associate Professor of Psychiatry and Pediatrics, Executive Director, Lifeline for Kids Program and Resilience Through Relationships Initiative, Department of Psychiatry, UMass Chan Medical School, North Worcester, Massachusetts, USA

NICOLE HEILBRON, PhD
Associate Professor, Department of Pediatrics, Duke University School of Medicine, Durham, North Carolina, USA

RACHEL B. HERBST, PhD
Associate Professor, Department of Pediatrics, University of Cincinnati College of Medicine, Director of Integrated Behavioral Health, General and Community Pediatrics,

Pediatric Psychologist, Division of Behavioral Medicine and Clinical Psychology, Cincinnati Children's Hospital Medical Center, Cincinnati, Ohio, USA

JENNIFER L. HUGHES, PhD, MPH
Associate Professor, Department of Psychiatry and Behavioral Health, The Ohio State University College of Medicine, Psychologist and Clinical Scholar, Behavioral Health Services, Division of Child and Family Psychiatry, Nationwide Children's Hospital, Columbus, Ohio, USA

KAY JOHNSON, MPH, EdM
President, Johnson Policy Consulting, Policy Lead, Nurture Connection, Hinesburg, Vermont, USA

CHRISTINA JOY, MD
Attending Psychiatrist, Department of Child and Adolescent Psychiatry and Behavioral Sciences, Children's Hospital of Philadelphia, Philadelphia, Pennsylvania, USA

CHUAN MEI LEE, MD, MA
Associate Professor, Department of Psychiatry and Behavioral Sciences, University of California San Francisco, Affiliated Scholar, Clinical Excellence Research Center, Stanford University School of Medicine, Stanford, California, USA

JOYCE Y. LEE, PhD
Assistant Professor, College of Social Work, The Ohio State University, Columbus, Ohio, USA

DAYNA LONG, MD
Professor, Department of Pediatrics, University of California, Ambassador, Nurture Connection, San Francisco, California, USA

GARY MASLOW, MD, MPH
Professor, Departments of Psychiatry and Behavioral Sciences, and Pediatrics, Duke University School of Medicine, Durham, North Carolina, USA

JESSICA M. McCLURE, PsyD
Associate Chief Population Health Officer, Office of Population Health, Division of Behavioral Medicine and Clinical Psychology, Cincinnati Children's Hospital Medical Center, Cincinnati, Ohio, USA

EMILY McTATE, PhD
Assistant Professor, Department of Pediatric and Adolescent Medicine, Mayo Clinic College of Medicine and Science, Pediatric Psychologist, Divison of Adolescent Psychiatry and Psychology, Mayo Clinic, Rochester, Minnesota, USA

ALAN MENDELSOHN, MD
Professor, Division of Developmental-Behavioral Pediatrics, Department of Pediatrics, NYU Grossman School of Medicine, New York, New York, USA

MARIE REILLY, MD
Instructor of Medicine, Division of Developmental Medicine, Boston Children's Hospital, Boston, Massachusetts, USA

LAURA P. RICHARDSON, MD, MPH
Professor, Department of Pediatrics, School of Medicine, University of Washington, Seattle, Washington, USA

ERIN ROBY, PhD
Assistant Professor, Division of Developmental-Behavioral Pediatrics, Department of Pediatrics, NYU Grossman School of Medicine, New York, New York, USA

DONNA A. RUCH, PhD
Principal Investigator, Center for Suicide Prevention and Research, The Abigail Wexner Research Institute, Nationwide Children's Hospital, Faculty member, Department of Pediatrics, The Ohio State University College of Medicine, Columbus, Ohio, USA

BARRY SARVET, MD
Professor and Chair, Department of Psychiatry, University of Massachusetts Medical School – Baystate, Springfield, Massachusetts, USA

PETER SZATMARI, MD, FRCPC, FRSC
Director of Cundill Centre for Child and Youth Depression, Center for Addiction and Mental Health, The Hospital for Sick Children, Emeritus Professor, Department of Psychiatry, Temerty Faculty of Medicine, University of Toronto, Toronto, Ontario, Canada

TRACY VAILLANCOURT, PhD, FRSC
Professor and Tier 1 Canada Research Chair, Professor in Counselling Psychology, Faculty of Education and School of Psychology, Faculty of Social Sciences, University of Ottawa, Ottawa, Ontario, Canada

BARBARA KEITH WALTER, PhD, MPH
Assistant Professor, Department of Psychiatry and Behavioral Sciences, Duke University School of Medicine, Durham, North Carolina, USA

CAROL WEITZMAN, MD
Associate Professor, Co-Director of the Autism Spectrum Center, Division of Developmental Medicine, Boston Children's Hospital, Boston, Massachusetts, USA

DAVID W. WILLIS, MD, FAAP
Founder and Director, Nurture Connection, Alexandria, Virginia; Professor of Pediatrics, Georgetown University, Georgetown University McCourt School of Public Policy, Center for Children and Families, Washington, DC, USA

LAWRENCE S. WISSOW, MD, MPH
Professor, Division of Child and Adolescent Psychiatry, Department of Psychiatry and Behavioral Sciences, School of Medicine, University of Washington, Seattle, Washington, USA

MELISSA A. YOUNG, PsyD
Attending Psychologist, Division of Behavioral Medicine and Clinical Psychology, Cincinnati Children's Hospital Medical Center, Assistant Professor, Department of Pediatrics, University of Cincinnati College of Medicine, Cincinnati, Ohio, USA

DANRUO ZHONG, PhD
Research Scientist, Division of Developmental-Behavioral Pediatrics, Department of Pediatrics, NYU Grossman School of Medicine, New York, New York, USA

Contents

Foreword: Declaration of a National Emergency in Child and Adolescent Mental Health: Where Do We Stand? xv

Tina L. Cheng

Preface: Innovative Approaches to Addressing Pediatric Mental Health xvii

Robert T. Ammerman and Craig A. Erickson

Epidemiology of Mental Health Challenges in Children and Adolescents 999

Ann H. Farrell, Peter Szatmari, and Tracy Vaillancourt

In this narrative review, we will discuss current understandings and evidence on child and adolescent mental health including epidemiologic research methods, prevalence rates of mental health difficulties before the coronavirus disease 2019 pandemic, changes in mental health challenges after the pandemic onset, and clinical implications.

Mental Health Screening and Measurement in Children and Adolescents 1013

Marie Reilly and Carol Weitzman

Approximately 20% of children experience a mental, emotional, or behavioral health problem each year and 40% will meet criteria for a disorder by the age of 18 years. The American Academy of Pediatrics now recommends global and domain-specific screening at every routine health maintenance visit starting in infancy. Based on US Preventative Services Task Force recommendations, anxiety screening should begin after the age of 8 years and depression and suicide risk screening after the age of 12 years. Screening should be combined with ongoing surveillance to ensure a comprehensive program to detect children with mental, emotional, and behavior problems.

Relational Health in Pediatrics 1027

David W. Willis, Dayna Long, and Kay Johnson

The American Academy of Pediatrics 2021 Policy Statement called for a paradigm shift that would prioritize clinical activities, rewrite research agendas, and realign collective advocacy by promoting relational health in partnership with communities and families. This seminal statement accelerated innovation toward high-performing medical homes, elevated family leadership and voices from family lived experiences, and advanced child health policies to move toward equity, child flourishing, and long-term well-being. More strengths-based, family-driven, and community connected practices among pediatric providers are essential to success. Early relational health approaches offer many opportunities for promoting social-emotional well-being, mental health, and flourishing.

Motivational Interviewing in Pediatric Mental Health 1047

Rachel B. Herbst, Alexandra M.S. Corley, Emily McTate, and Julie M. Gettings

Although many pediatric clinicians have familiarity with motivational interviewing (MI), they may have limited awareness of how it can benefit mental and behavioral health assessment and management. This article describes the spirit, tasks, and skills of MI. Cases illustrate the application of MI to common presentations of mental health concerns in pediatric primary care. These examples provide concrete guidance on how to navigate barriers to applying MI and underscore how MI aligns with the unique opportunities and values of primary care, including longitudinal relationships, opportunities to partner with families in shared decision-making, and valuing culturally-responsive, patient-centered care.

Practice-Based Models of Pediatric Mental Health Care 1059

Chuan Mei Lee, Jayme Congdon, Christina Joy, and Barry Sarvet

Pediatric primary care is widely available in the United States and can help address the growing public health crisis in child and adolescent mental health by providing integrated behavioral health services. This article provides an overview of 3 common models of behavioral health integration in pediatric primary care settings: 1) the Child Psychiatry Access Program model, 2) the Primary Care Behavioral Health model, and 3) the Collaborative Care Model. Pediatric primary care practices may evaluate the different features of each model before adopting an approach for integration and consider tailoring it to their practice environments.

Integrated Behavioral Health: A Guide to Practical Implementation 1073

Jessica M. McClure and Melissa A. Young

Integrating behavioral health providers in primary care settings is an effective model for increasing access to mental and behavioral health services for youth. Resources and subject matter experts can be leveraged by pediatric practices to identify the components of a successful model and to support implementation in community practices. Integrated behavioral health approaches vary in scope and components of the models can be selected and implemented to meet the needs of each practice and the patient population served.

Pediatric Mental Health Prevention Programs in Primary Care 1087

Yu Chen, Danruo Zhong, Erin Roby, Caitlin Canfield, and Alan Mendelsohn

Children's mental health problems are pressing social, economic, and public health concerns in the U.S. While pediatric primary care offers important venues to integrate mental health services for children and their families, new challenges, including widening educational, economic, and health disparities in the context of structural racism and COVID-related social isolation, underscore the need for innovative approaches. The authors reviewed 6 innovative methods in pediatric care that have helped address these issues and amplify intervention efforts focused on children's mental health. Limitations and future directions for research and clinical practice in pediatric mental health services are also discussed.

Trauma-Informed Strategies in Pediatric Primary Care 1101

Heather Forkey and Jessica Griffin

Child trauma, particularly within the context of the caregiving relationship, can have profound impacts on health, thus pediatric clinicians have a crucial role in recognizing and responding to trauma. Yet, trauma-informed care (TIC) is often described by its guiding principles rather than an approach to implementation. TIC requires the pediatric clinician to not only be familiar with the physiology of trauma, but actively promote resilience and employ strategies for primary prevention, secondary response and tertiary treatment of trauma. This study covers practical approaches to care that allow for promoting resilience, and the recognition, diagnosis and management of trauma.

Evidence-Based Youth Suicide Prevention and Intervention in Pediatric Primary Care Settings 1119

Donna A. Ruch, Jennifer L. Hughes, Jeffrey A. Bridge, and Cynthia A. Fontanella

Suicide is a leading cause of death in youth. Evidence highlights the importance of identifying youth at risk for suicide in pediatric primary care, and suggests this is a crucial setting for improving youth mental health. The American Academy of Pediatrics recommends primary care providers not only screen and assess for suicide risk, but also become educated on how to better manage certain mental health conditions. This article discusses the epidemiology of youth suicide in the United States and describes evidence-based strategies and innovative practices for suicide prevention in pediatric primary care including suicide risk screening, assessment, intervention, and follow-up care.

Addressing Mental Health and Social Needs in Tandem to Promote Health Equity 1141

Chidiogo Anyigbo, Sarah J. Beal, Joyce Y. Lee, and Laura M. Gottlieb

Compelling evidence shows that social risks and mental health are intertwined. Pediatric clinicians can maximize the effectiveness of interventions that address mental health concerns by incorporating social risks and social needs screening and interventions. Approaches that elevate the interconnectedness of social risks and mental health require (a) an understanding of the multi-level contextual factors that contribute to patient and family functioning; and (b) a culturally responsive and multidisciplinary clinical practice that targets contextual factors. Supporting families to see the value of concurrently addressing social and mental health needs may be an important step to amplify clinical practice changes.

Innovative Approaches to Addressing Pediatric Mental Health: Digital Technologies in Pediatric Primary Care 1151

Gary Maslow, Richard Chung, Nicole Heilbron, and Barbara Keith Walter

Digital technologies can be used at multiple levels to support the mental health care of children including (1) health system/health care provider level; (2) patient–provider interface; (3) patient-facing consumer applications; and (4) new technology, including artificial intelligence. At each of these levels, these novel technologies may lead to care improvements but also may have risks. This review provides an overview of each of innovations across the digital landscape.

A "Next Generation" of Pediatric Mental Health Systems **1165**

Lawrence S. Wissow and Laura P. Richardson

An optimistic view of the future child/youth mental health system is that it will be oriented toward prevention and shaped by innovations in early detection and treatment of functional problems, coupled with the power of digital technology to provide new ways to help individuals and families monitor their well-being and seek or agree to help as it is needed. These innovations will be deployed within a community-based health care system, centered on primary care that fully implements ideas about continuity and comprehensiveness (including social determinants, substance use, and multigenerational care) that have been around for decades.

PEDIATRIC CLINICS OF NORTH AMERICA

FORTHCOMING ISSUES

February 2025
Challenges of Pediatric Practice in Rural America
Mary C. Ottolini, *Editor*

April 2025
Social Media and Pediatric Mental Health
Paul E. Weigle and Erin L. Belfort, *Editors*

June 2025
Recognizing and Responding to Child Maltreatment
Allison M. Jackson, *Editor*

RECENT ISSUES

October 2024
Obesity
Gitanjali Srivastava and Eliana M. Perrin, *Editors*

August 2024
Adolescent Medicine: Important Updates after the COVID-19 Pandemic
Renata Arrington Sanders and Errol L. Fields, *Editors*

June 2024
Pandemic Planning in Pediatrics
Yvonne A. Maldonado, Steven E. Krug and Erica Y. Popovsky, *Editors*

Foreword

Declaration of a National Emergency in Child and Adolescent Mental Health: Where Do We Stand?

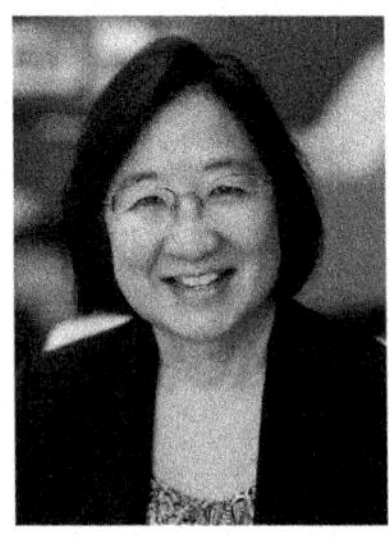

Tina L. Cheng, MD, MPH
Consulting Editor

In late 2021, the American Academy of Pediatrics, American Academy of Child and Adolescent Psychiatry and Children's Hospital Association declared a national emergency in child and adolescent mental health. Citing soaring rates of mental health issues and inequities from structural racism, it was a clear call to action.

Successful action to address this issue relies on several principles. First, upstream prevention and health promotion are key. While there is a shortage of child psychiatric hospital beds, building more beds is not the long-term solution. Understanding the antecedents of mental and behavioral conditions and ensuring mental and emotional well-being are essential.

Second, health care will not solve the mental health crisis alone. The health care system must partner with schools, social services, juvenile justice, community agencies, childcare, and other sectors in partnership to achieve our shared goal of child well-being and success.

Third, health equity and community cocreation and codesign must be central to ensure that all children and adolescents thrive. The voices of children, youth, and families are essential to understand and address the biases and barriers that currently exist.

Fourth, the workforce supporting the needs of children, adolescents, and families must be strengthened and expanded. Ensuring a trained and accessible workforce that uses evidence-based practices and measuring outcomes are critical components for progress. Training additional workforce members in supporting the mental and

Pediatr Clin N Am 71 (2024) xv–xvi
https://doi.org/10.1016/j.pcl.2024.08.001

behavioral health of children (eg, primary care clinicians, behavioral health specialists in schools) is also needed.

Finally, we need innovation to build a system of support and health care for children and adolescents. Instead of siloed initiatives and Band-Aid solutions, new ideas and a coordinated system that supports child thriving and care are urgently needed.

In light of a national emergency, this *Pediatric Clinics of North America* issue focuses on child and adolescent mental health. It documents where we stand, reviews progress, and charts new directions. While there has been progress, this issue is a call to action.

Tina L. Cheng, MD, MPH
Cincinnati Children's Hospital Medical Center
University of Cincinnati
Cincinnati Children's Research Foundation
3333 Burnet Avenue, MLC 3016
Cincinnati, OH 45229-3026, USA

E-mail address:
Tina.cheng@cchmc.org

Preface

Innovative Approaches to Addressing Pediatric Mental Health

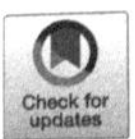

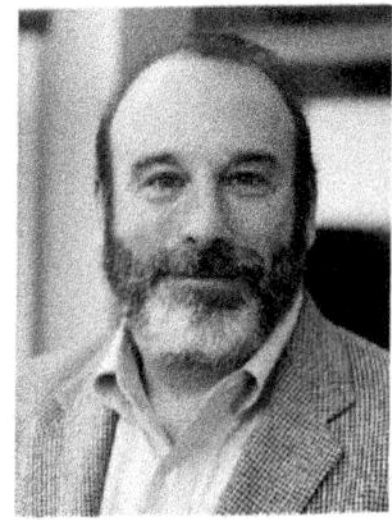

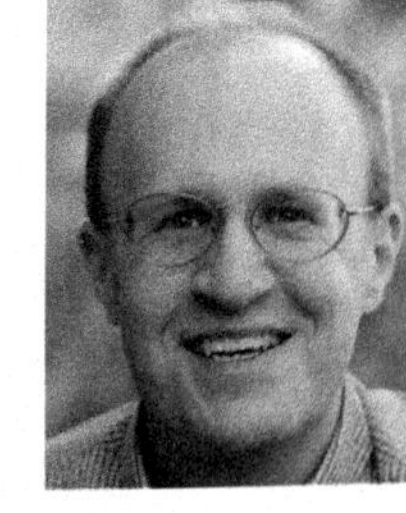

Robert T. Ammerman, PhD Craig A. Erickson, MD
Editors

It is widely acknowledged that there is a mental health epidemic among children and adolescents. Recent epidemiologic studies document that over 1 in 3 children and adolescents develop significant symptoms of a psychiatric disorder, and for many their conditions will continue into adulthood.[1] These alarming statistics increased during the COVID-19 pandemic, focusing a bright spotlight on what is clearly a national crisis.[2] Primary care pediatricians are on the frontline of addressing this problem. With near universal contact with children and families, primary care pediatricians are typically the first to identify emotional and behavioral health concerns. Until recently, referral to outside specialists was the sole option when encountering psychiatric conditions in need of evaluation and treatment. This has changed in the past two decades, as new models and strategies to support the emotional and behavioral health of children in primary care settings have emerged.

Given the shortage of mental health specialists, primary care pediatricians are often called upon to assume the management and care of children and adolescents with behavioral health conditions. The primary care setting is, in many ways, well-positioned to promote behavioral health and support children and adolescents with psychiatric disorders and their families. The holistic approach to care and support of healthy development and well-being makes primary care settings appealing locations for prevention and treatment. By building the capacity of primary care offices to support behavioral health, access to care is expanded, and health disparities can be reduced. Primary ... n essential resource as we develop new strategies and systems to ... al health crisis in children and adolescents.[3]

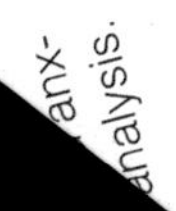

(2024) xvii–xix
/j.pcl.2024.07.038
iblished by Elsevier Inc.

In this issue of *Pediatric Clinics of North America*, we have asked leading experts in the field to describe some of these new approaches that are transforming both primary care and the wider mental health care system. Farrell and colleagues first describe what we know about the epidemiology of mental health problems and in children and adolescents, including the recent increases in prevalence. Reilly and Weltzman then review screening for emotional and behavioral issues, as early detection can lead to more responsive interventions and improved outcomes. Willis and colleagues (relational health) and Herbst and colleagues (motivational interviewing) describe important strategies for pediatricians to support behavioral health in their patients. Sarvet and Lee and McClure and Young describe practice-based models and integrated behavioral health approaches to mental health care, respectively. Chen and colleagues review the embedding of prevention programs in primary care, utilizing this setting to promote healthy behavioral development and reduce the incidence of psychiatric disorders. Forkey and Griffin discuss trauma-informed care of children and families, an essential aspect of clinical practice for those who have experienced abuse, neglect, and adversity. Ruch and colleagues discuss suicide prevention and intervention programs in primary care. Anyigbo and colleagues describe how primary care can support families with social needs. Maslow and Chung review the use of digital technologies and platforms to address mental health concerns. Finally, Wissow and Richardson provide guidance and suggestions to improve the mental health system, leveraging the opportunities and resources of the primary care setting.

This is an exciting time for innovation and new ideas in providing behavioral health care in the primary care setting. The articles in this issue document the tremendous progress that has been made. However, this is a foundation on which to build. In the coming decades, we look forward to the development of novel and effective approaches to support children and families.

DISCLOSURES

The authors have no conflicts of interest to disclose.

Robert T. Ammerman, PhD
Cincinnati Children's Hospital Medical Center
University of Cincinnati College of Medicine
3333 Burnett Avenue
Cincinnati, OH 45229-3026, USA

Craig A. Erickson, MD
Cincinnati Children's Hospital Medical Center
University of Cincinnati College of Medicine
3333 Burnett Avenue
Cincinnati, OH 45229-3026, USA

E-mail addresses:
robert.ammerman@cchmc.org (R.T. Ammerman)
craig.erickson@cchmc.org (C.A. Erickson)

REFERENCES

1. Racine N, McArthur BA, Cooke JE, et al. Global prevalence of depressive [illegible] iety symptoms in children and adolescents during COVID-19: a meta[illegible] JAMA Pediatr 2021;175(11):1142.

2. Alizadeh S, Shahrousvand S, Sepandi M, et al. Prevalence of anxiety, depression and post-traumatic stress disorder symptoms in children and adolescents during the COVID-19 pandemic: a systematic review and meta-analysis. J Public Health 2023;1–16. https://doi.org/10.1007/s10389-023-02168-w.
3. Sorter M, Stark LJ, Glauser T, et al. Addressing the pediatric mental health crisis: moving from a reactive to a proactive system of care. J Pediatr 2024; 265:113479.

Epidemiology of Mental Health Challenges in Children and Adolescents

Ann H. Farrell, PhD[a,*], Peter Szatmari, MD, FRCPC, FRSC[b,c], Tracy Vaillancourt, PhD, FRSC[d]

KEYWORDS

- Children • Adolescents • Mental health • Population-based • Longitudinal
- Meta-analyses • Epidemiology • COVID-19 pandemic

KEY POINTS

- Longitudinal, population-based, and meta-analytic studies reveal that mental health challenges in children and adolescents were a significant public health problem before the pandemic.
- Since the coronavirus disease 2019 pandemic, mental health challenges including anxiety, depression, suicide attempts, and eating disorders among children and adolescents have increased more than expected based on prepandemic estimates.
- Increased efforts are needed for mental health screening in high-risk child and adolescent populations.

INTRODUCTION

The developmental periods of childhood and adolescence reflect a time of immense biological, psychological, cognitive, and social changes. These periods also coincide with the onset of 50% to 75% of mental health disorders.[1,2] Meta-analytic findings indicate that the peak age of onset for mental health disorders is 14.5 years, with 48.4% of onset occurring before age 18 years[3] and 13.4% of children and adolescents experiencing serious mental health challenges at one point in time.[4] These trends are concerning given that mental health challenges can seriously interrupt critical developmental milestones occurring during childhood and adolescence.[5,6] Moreover, mental health disorders are the leading cause of disease-related burden worldwide[7] in this population and are associated with long-term adverse outcomes across the

[a] Department of Child and Youth Studies, Brock University, 1812 Sir Isaac Brock Way, St Catharines, Ontario L2S 3A1, Canada; [b] Center for Addiction and Mental Health, Hospital for Sick Children, 80 Workman Way, Toronto, Ontario M6J 1H4, Canada; [c] Department of Psychiatry, Temerty Faculty of Medicine, University of Toronto, Toronto, Ontario, Canada; [d] Counselling Psychology, Faculty of Education and School of Psychology, Faculty of Social Sciences, University of Ottawa, 145 Jean-Jacques-Lussier, Ontario K1N 6N5, Canada
* Corresponding author.
E-mail address: afarrell@brocku.ca

Pediatr Clin N Am 71 (2024) 999–1011
https://doi.org/10.1016/j.pcl.2024.07.009 pediatric.theclinics.com

lifespan including the continuity of mental health challenges, death by suicide, poorer academic achievement, and lower economic advancement.[8–11]

Findings from epidemiologic studies and meta-analyses indicate that mental health challenges among children and adolescents were a serious concern before the coronavirus disease 2019 (COVID-19) pandemic.[4] Studies that have emerged since the pandemic onset indicate that child and adolescent mental health challenges have continued, if not increased, for many individuals. Accordingly, researchers and practitioners have recommended investigating mental health challenges across childhood (ages 12 years and younger), adolescence (ages 13–18 years), and young adulthood (ages 18–25 years) to capture a thorough understanding of the epidemiology and developmental course of mental health difficulties.[7] These scientific investigations can contribute to effective evidence-based practices to prevent mental health challenges and adverse outcomes. In this narrative review, we will discuss current understandings and evidence on child and adolescent mental health including epidemiologic research methods, prevalence rates of mental health challenges before the COVID-19 pandemic, changes in mental health difficulties after the COVID-19 pandemic onset, and clinical implications.

EPIDEMIOLOGIC RESEARCH METHODS IN CHILD AND ADOLESCENT MENTAL HEALTH

To comprehensively understand the epidemiology of child and adolescent mental health challenges, rigorous research methodology is needed. Child and adolescent mental health challenges are the result of multiple independent and interacting risk factors. From a developmental psychopathology framework, transactions across biological, genetic, individual, social, and environmental factors can contribute to the mental health challenges among children and adolescents.[12] Similar transactional pathways can lead to different outcomes (ie, multifinality), and different pathways can lead to similar outcomes (ie, equifinality). Results across large-scale, longitudinal and population-based studies are needed to examine these pathways to identify modifiable processes. Robust methodologies contribute to understanding the developmental patterns seen on average across childhood and adolescence and how these developmental patterns are heterogeneous across subpopulations of individuals.

Systematic reviews and meta-analyses are informative for understanding the epidemiology of mental health challenges in children and adolescents by collating all studies on a given topic. Meta-analyses provide an additional summary effect size that reflects a more precise indicator than single studies of whether a finding is, on average, robust.[13] Meta-analyses also allow for examining heterogeneity of effects across different studies and include a systematic assessment of risks of bias (eg, publication bias) and moderators of effect sizes (eg, study methodology and sample characteristics). Meta-analyses on population-based longitudinal or birth cohort studies that follow the same individuals across time are the gold standard for understanding the development of mental health problems, whereas randomized control trials are the gold standard for studies of causation.[14]

Longitudinal studies allow for examining change in population-based samples. Variable-centered analyses allow for examining development in an overall sample (see Brittain and Vaillancourt,[14] for a review). One type of variable-centered analysis is known as a latent growth curve, which allows for examining how a given mental health challenge changes or remains stable across time (eg, linear increase or decrease, curvilinear or quadratic increase or decrease). Another type of variable-centered analysis is a cascade model, which allows for examining the temporal priority of risk factors and outcomes of mental health challenges. This temporal priority can reveal whether the association between mental health difficulties and risk factors are unidirectional or bidirectional across development. For example, in a sample of 695 Canadian individuals followed across ages 10 to 14 years, a symptoms-driven pathway was supported, with internalizing problems consistently predicting subsequent bullying victimization.[15] A third type of variable-centered analysis involves separating between-person associations (eg, a child's anxiety relative to others' anxiety) from within-person associations (eg, a child's anxiety relative to their own anxiety) across development.[16] For example, increases within an individual's generalized anxiety symptoms consistently predicted that individual's increases in depression symptoms across adolescence in a Canadian sample.[17]

Where there is evidence of heterogeneity in change over time, person-centered analyses in longitudinal studies allow for investigating distinct patterns of change among subpopulations of individuals. In other words, rather than running a latent growth curve on a given mental health challenge for the overall sample, person-centered analyses allow for finding subgroups within the sample that follow distinct growth patterns across time. For example, in one study of 701 Canadians, most youth were low on anxiety symptoms across ages 10 to 18 years (47.2%), but smaller groups reflected moderate (37.3%) and high increasing levels (15.5%), with the latter group being over 15 and 19 times more likely to be diagnosed with social anxiety disorder and have a depressive episode, respectively, across ages 19 to 22 years compared to the low group.[10] Pooling effect sizes across these longitudinal studies in a meta-analysis can help reveal overall and heterogeneous robust developmental patterns of mental health challenges including change, risk factors, and outcomes. These longitudinal designs are especially informative for understanding the impact of the COVID-19 pandemic on mental health, which requires a baseline assessment of mental health before the pandemic in the same sample of individuals.[18,19]

In the absence of longitudinal studies, meta-analyses with large representative samples of population-based studies that are cross-sectional, or incidence studies are also informative for understanding the prevalence and correlates of mental disorders in children and adolescents. Many of the meta-analyses that provide information on the prevalence and age of onset of mental health challenges in children and adolescents are based on population-based studies. For example, a meta-analysis of 192 epidemiologic studies (n = 708,561) by Solmi and colleagues[3] examined the age of onset of mental disorders based on a combination of cross-sectional studies (n = 150), incidence studies (n = 27), and birth cohort studies (n = 15). The researchers found evidence for a developmental chronology for the peak age of onset of mental disorders. This chronology started with neurodevelopmental disorders (5.5 years) and anxiety and fear-related disorders (5.5 years), followed by obsessive-compulsive related disorders (14.5 years), feeding or eating disorders (15.5 years), disorders due to substance use or addictive behavior (19.5 years), schizophrenia-spectrum and primary psychotic disorders (20.5 years), personality disorders (20.5 years), and mood disorders (20.5 years). As suggested by several other researchers (eg, Kieling and colleagues[7]), these developmental trends demonstrate the importance of examining multiple age groups across childhood and adolescence.

CHILD AND ADOLESCENT MENTAL HEALTH BEFORE THE CORONAVIRUS DISEASE 2019 PANDEMIC

Prevalence rates of child and adolescent mental health disorders were high before the COVID-19 pandemic. Meta-analytic findings demonstrated that across studies conducted between 1985 and 2012, the prevalence of mental disorders among individuals aged between 5 and 18 years was 13.4%.[4] Prevalence rates can vary by measurement tools (eg, self-report and clinical interviews), by informants (eg, self-report, parent-report, teacher, and clinician), and by definition (eg, symptoms vs disorder, whether impairment is part of the definition of disorder). For some of the more common forms of disorders, prevalence rates were 6.5% for any anxiety disorder, 3.4% for attention deficit hyperactivity disorder (ADHD), 2.6% for any depressive disorder, 2.1% for conduct disorder, and 5.7% for any disruptive disorder. Recent prepandemic evidence also supports similar prevalence rates. Prepandemic data from the Global Burden of Disease Study, based on 1742 data sources across 143 countries, revealed that 1 in 10 individuals between the ages 5 to 24 years had at least one mental disorder.[7] These data also showed that the average prevalence of mental disorders was 11.63% and when broken down by age included 6.81% for ages 5 to 9 years, 12.41% for ages 10 to 14 years, 13.96% for ages 15 to 19 years, and 13.63% for ages 20 to 24 years. Consistent with previous meta-analyses, the highest prevalence rates found were for anxiety disorders (3.35%). Sex differences were also evident for most disorders, although they varied by the disorder (eg, higher rates of anxiety disorders for girls and higher rates of ADHD for boys). In another recent study using electronic health records between 2010 and 2023 of individuals aged younger than 21 years, Elia and colleagues[20] found that 19.8% of individuals without adverse childhood experiences (ACEs) and 20.4% of individuals with ACEs had a lifetime prevalence of mental health disorders and/or symptoms. Evidence also indicated that prevalence rates increased from 10.6% in 2010 to 15.1% in 2023, with the highest rate of 15.4% occurring 1 year before the COVID-19 pandemic in 2019. Risks for experiencing a mental health disorder or symptom was higher for adolescents (vs younger ages), boys (vs girls), and White individuals (vs other races/ethnicities). See **Table 1** for a summary of the prevalence rates for common mental health disorders in children and adolescents presented by Polanczyk and colleagues,[4] Kieling and colleagues,[7] and Elia and colleagues.[20]

In addition to prevalence rates of mental disorders in children and adolescents, it is also important to understand lifetime prevalence rates that include adults. In a study by McGrath and colleagues[21] based on cross-sectional epidemiologic data from

Table 1
Summary of prevalence rates for common mental health disorders in children and adolescents presented by Polanczyk et al,[4] Elia et al,[20] and Kieling et al[7]

	Prevalence (%)		
	Polanczyk et al,[4] 2015	**Elia et al,[20] 2023[a]**	**Kieling et al,[7] 2024**
Any anxiety disorder	6.5	5.81	3.35
Attention deficit hyperactivity disorder (ADHD)	3.4	-	2.23
Any depressive disorder	2.6	3.45[b]	1.84
Conduct disorder	2.1	1.99[c]	1.59
Any mental disorder	13.4	20.36	11.63

[a] We calculated rates based on prevalence per 1000 patients presented by Elia et al.[20]
[b] Mood disorders.
[c] Disruptive behavior disorders.

2001 to 2022 across individuals aged 18 years or older from 17 high-income countries and 12 low or middle-income countries, the lifetime prevalence of any mental disorder was 28.6% for men and 29.8% for women. In this study, participants were asked about their current and retrospective (ie, earliest age including childhood) mental health symptoms. For men, the most prevalent mental disorders were major depressive disorder and alcohol use disorder, whereas for women they were major depressive disorder and specific phobia. Prevalence rates among adults are informative given the continuity of mental disorders from childhood to adulthood.[10] Children and adolescents are also nested within families with adult caregivers that may also be experiencing mental health challenges, which in turn are likely to impact the mental health of these children and adolescents.[18]

Evidence also supports that prepandemic prevalence of mental health disorders differed by several key demographic factors. A systematic review of 55 studies between 1990 and 2011 on individuals aged between 4 and 18 years showed that children and adolescents from lower socioeconomic backgrounds were 2 to 3 times more likely to develop mental health challenges than peers from higher socioeconomic backgrounds.[22] The negative association between socioeconomic status and mental health challenges was stronger among children aged 12 years and younger relative to children aged over 12 years. However, the strength of association between socioeconomic status and mental health challenges by sex was inconsistent as patterns varied by type of mental health difficulty. Several common methods of assessing socioeconomic status were included in this systematic review such as household income, parental education level, and parental occupation status, further demonstrating the importance of adult caregivers in impacting child and adolescent mental health.

Minority status in other demographic factors such as race/ethnicity and gender identity can also play a role in mental health challenges. In a systematic review of 13 studies, higher proportions of same race students in schools across the United States, United Kingdom, and Netherlands were associated with better overall mental health, but schools with greater racial diversity did not demonstrate significant advantages to mental health.[23] In another systematic review of studies conducted between 2000 and 2020, racial minority individuals aged between 11 and 22 years in the United States were less likely to use mental health services than White individuals, with barriers to services including socioeconomic disadvantage and cultural factors.[24] Thus, socioeconomic disadvantage often intersects with other demographic factors such as racial/ethnic minority status.[18] For gender and sexual identity, a meta-analysis of studies conducted until January 2020 including individuals aged 12 to 25 years revealed that the prevalence of victimization and mental health difficulties among lesbian, gay, bisexual, transgender, and queer (LGBTQ+) individuals with experiences of self-harm or suicide (ideation or behavior) were 3.74 and 2.67 times higher, respectively, when matched to cisgender and heterosexual peers.[25]

An additional aspect of investigating child and adolescent mental health challenges is to recognize the co-occurrence of mental and physical health challenges. In a systematic review of 431 studies on individuals aged 18 years and younger, evidence supported the multimorbidity of mental health disorders and physical health illnesses. Data were primarily cross-sectional and indicated that most research supported the multimorbidity of mental health disorders such as anxiety, mood, and attention disorders, and to a lesser degree behavioral disorders (eg, conduct disorder) with physical illnesses such as epilepsy, asthma, allergies, chronic pain, and diabetes mellitus.[26] Thus, for a comprehensive understanding of the epidemiology of mental health challenges, the connection among internalizing problems, externalizing problems, and neurodevelopmental disorders with one another and with physical health must be understood, especially in light of the increased risk for physical illness after the onset of the COVID-19 pandemic.

CHILD AND ADOLESCENT MENTAL HEALTH AFTER THE CORONAVIRUS DISEASE 2019 PANDEMIC ONSET

The onset of the COVID-19 pandemic resulted in extreme changes to daily routine to prevent the spread of severe acute respiratory syndrome coronavirus 2, including lockdowns, social distancing, and cancellation of in-person school and community events. As a result, a significant number of studies have been dedicated to understanding the impact of the pandemic on child and adolescent mental health. Studies on internalizing symptoms (eg, difficulty with regulating emotions or mood; depression, anxiety, and somatization[15]) were common, given these symptoms are some of the most prevalent forms of mental health challenges experienced by children and adolescents. Early pandemic studies were primarily cross-sectional (ie, mental health assessed only after pandemic onset) or retrospective (ie, asking individuals to recall how their mental health has changed since before the pandemic), preventing a clear understanding of true change in mental health.[18] Nevertheless, meta-analyses based on these studies are informative in revealing the overall patterns of child and adolescent mental health within the first year of the pandemic.

Racine and colleagues[27] conducted the first meta-analysis of 29 studies from the first year of the COVID-19 pandemic (until March 2021) to examine child and adolescent depression and anxiety symptoms. The prevalence of clinically elevated depression symptoms was 25.2% and anxiety symptoms was 20.5%, with these prevalence rates being significantly higher among girls, older individuals, and in studies conducted later in the pandemic. These findings were significant in demonstrating that the prevalence rates of clinically elevated depression and anxiety symptoms had doubled during the first year of the pandemic in comparison to before the pandemic. In a more recent meta-analysis of cross-sectional and longitudinal studies conducted between 2020 and December 2022, Alizadeh and colleagues[28] found that the prevalence of anxiety symptoms was 26% and the prevalence of depression symptoms and post-traumatic stress disorder symptoms were each 23%. Anxiety prevalence was highest in Europe (43.2%), whereas depression prevalence was highest in North America (35.4%).

As the pandemic continued, meta-analyses examining longitudinal pandemic studies emerged. Madigan and colleagues[29] examined 53 longitudinal studies capturing 40,807 children and adolescents across 12 countries to examine depression and anxiety symptoms between 2020 and May 2022. An increase in depression symptoms was found (standardized mean change [SMC] = 0.26). An increase in anxiety symptoms were also found, although to a lesser degree than depression (SMC = 0.10). In addition, compared to prepandemic levels, increases in depression symptoms during the pandemic were seen among girls (SMC = 0.32), individuals from mid-to-high income backgrounds (SMC = 0.35), and in North America (SMC = 0.25) and Europe (SMC = 0.35). These latter demographic findings contrasted the predominant assumption that affluent children and adolescents fared well during the pandemic. Instead, these findings highlight that affluent children and adolescents, in particular adolescent girls, should be supported during the pandemic along with underrepresented and marginalized individuals. One suggested mechanism contributing to the increases in internalizing symptoms during the pandemic has been the lack of prepandemic levels of support that were available due to social isolation. Evidence from a systematic review revealed that loneliness increased in longitudinal studies among children and adolescents during the pandemic, was associated with depression symptoms and anxiety symptoms, and moderated increases in suicide risk.[30] Considering that the pandemic-related social restrictions likely increased feelings of social isolation and loneliness, the absence of positive social relationships appeared to contribute to mental health challenges such as internalizing symptoms and suicide risk.

Suicide attempts were a significant area of concern after the COVID-19 pandemic onset. Madigan and colleagues[31] conducted a meta-analysis on 42 studies conducted between 2020 and December 2022 that had data before and after the pandemic onset. This meta-analysis captured 11.1 million child and adolescent emergency department visits for suicide ideation, self-harm, and attempted suicide across 18 countries. Significant increases were found compared to prepandemic levels in attempted suicide (rate ratio [RR] = 1.22) and suicide ideation (RR = 1.08). Like the results on internalizing symptoms, the increases found for a combination of attempted suicide and suicide ideation were stronger in girls and older individuals. A study using a large database of electronic health records from 5 large medical centers in the New York City metropolitan area support findings by Madigan and colleagues[31] within the waves of the pandemic. Levine and colleagues[32] examined rates of mental health-related emergency department visits among individuals aged 5 to 17 years across the first 5 waves of COVID-19 (up to June 2022). Mental health-related emergency department visits were significantly higher at each pandemic wave than prepandemic rates, with the highest rates at wave 2, which was also the longest wave duration (ie, August 2020–June 2021). Increased visits were seen for eating disorders at all waves, anxiety disorders in all but 1 wave, substance use disorders in all but 2 waves, and depressive disorders and suicidality/self-harm at wave 2. Increased visits were also seen among girls, adolescents, individuals from Asian backgrounds, and individuals from higher socioeconomic backgrounds. Similarly, in a recent meta-analysis by Madigan and colleagues,[33] there was a 54% increase in eating disorder-related emergency department visits during the pandemic compared to before the pandemic, with this effect being more pronounced among girls (relative to boys) and adolescents (relative to children).

Several meta-analyses and systematic reviews examined the prevalence of additional externalizing symptoms (eg, difficulty with regulating behavior; attention, conduct, and aggression problems[15]) in children and adolescents. Rogers and MacLean[34] conducted a meta-analysis of 18 studies conducted until November 2022 on ADHD symptoms in individuals aged 3 to 18 years across 10 countries; 12 studies were longitudinal and 6 studies were retrospective. Longitudinal studies needed to have data from before and after the pandemic onset, whereas retrospective studies needed to have data that were retrospective before the pandemic and concurrent during the pandemic. A small significant increase in ADHD symptoms was found ($d = 0.27$), with no significant differences between study design (ie, longitudinal vs retrospective), or by sex or age. A recently published population-based study by Antoniou and colleagues[35] on all residents of Ontario, Canada, aged 24 years and younger support these developmental trends. Using health databases, stimulant prescription dispensing was compared before the pandemic (January 2013–March 2020) to after the pandemic onset (April 2020–June 2022). Early in the pandemic until May 2020, there was a significant decrease in prescription dispensing, followed by a return to prepandemic levels by June 2021, then an increase. Overall, the rate of stimulant prescription dispensing among individuals increased 62.6% from 2013 to 2022, with significant increases among girls/women, individuals aged 20 to 24 years, and individuals from higher socioeconomic backgrounds. Significant decreases were found among boys/men and individuals aged 0 to 4 years and 5 to 9 years. The researchers concluded that additional research is needed to ensure that stimulants are being used appropriately, rather than for nonmedical purposes.

Substance use has further been examined in a systematic review by Layman and colleagues[36] who reviewed 49 studies (20 longitudinal and 29 cross-sectional) on individuals aged 24 years and younger conducted until February 2022. Most studies reflected a decrease in the prevalence of substances (eg, alcohol, cannabis, tobacco, and e-cigarette/vaping), except for 3 studies that found an increase in other and unspecified types of substance use. However, using data from the Centers for Disease Control and Prevention WONDER database,[37] researchers recently highlighted that although illicit drug use has declined among adolescents, overdose-related deaths (eg, due to opioids) has doubled among adolescents aged between 14 and 18 years in the United States between August 2019 and March 2020.[38] Moreover, some of the highest rates were evident among some racial/ethnic minority adolescents.[39] There is also evidence of heterogeneity in substance use. Among Canadian individuals aged 14 to 28 years, most individuals demonstrated low and stable substance use across the early stages of the pandemic until October 2020 (58.8%), but smaller groups of individuals reported somewhat higher (27.6%) and highest (13.6%) stable levels of substance use.[40]

Similar to the overall declines seen for substance use, a recent comprehensive narrative review revealed that the prevalence of school bullying reflected initial declines early in the pandemic.[41] This effect was predominately found in countries and regions with a greater number of pandemic mitigation social restrictions. However, countries and regions with fewer restrictions reflected increases in bullying prevalence rates. These findings again provide evidence for the importance of social relationships in mental health problems, in particular the heterogeneity and multiple developmental pathways experienced by children and adolescents.[12] Social restrictions can contribute to feelings of loneliness for some individuals, but they can also reduce experiences of negative in-person social relationships (ie, bullying) for other individuals. The presence of negative in-person social relationships can also contribute to adverse mental health. Indeed, it has been well established that experiencing bullying victimization is associated with a host of mental health problems including depression, anxiety, and increased risk for suicidality (see McDougall and Vaillancourt[42] and Moore and colleagues,[43] for a review). Given that few longitudinal studies have examined change in bullying from before to after the pandemic onset, additional evidence is needed to understand whether bullying has, in fact, changed due to the pandemic.

Together, these meta-analyses, systematic reviews, and comprehensive narrative reviews indicate that many internalizing symptoms (ie, depression and anxiety), eating disorders, and suicide attempts have increased on average from before to during the pandemic. There is also evidence of increases in some forms of externalizing symptoms (ie, ADHD) and possibly overdoses. However, other types of mental health challenges like substance use have declined or have mixed evidence (ie, bullying).

Given that it has been 4 years since the pandemic onset, an increasing number of high-quality and robust population-based, incidence ratio, and longitudinal studies on the impact of the COVID-19 pandemic on child and adolescent mental health are emerging. Integrating evidence from these recent studies with evidence from prepandemic studies will provide a more thorough, comprehensive understanding on the epidemiology of child and adolescent mental health challenges and how they are evolving across time. These contributions will further help prevent, intervene, and predict mental health challenges to provide a proactive and evidence-based approach to support children and adolescents, including among individuals at highest risk.

CLINICAL IMPLICATIONS

It is important to address the inequity in mental health across the population by committing to child and adolescent mental health recovery, which should include efforts to reduce stressors that promote poor mental health (eg, poverty, bullying victimization, discrimination, and poor parental mental health). A critical challenge to the increase in the number of children and adolescents affected is that there was little capacity to manage this issue clinically before the pandemic. In fact, before the pandemic only 20% of children and adolescents with mental health challenges received services, and those that did, tended to have more severe impairing mental disorders.[44,45] Moreover, most services were provided through schools,[46] which were closed for 1.9 billion children and adolescents in the first year of the pandemic.[47] To better manage this mental health crisis, innovative solutions are needed. Vaillancourt and colleagues[48] suggested that there should be targeted screening among high-risk groups and that diagnosis and treatment services should be delivered in environments where children and adolescents can easily access, such as primary health care settings, or better yet, school settings. They further suggested that school-based mental health strategies ought to focus on health and wellness promotion at the universal level and that, when needed, these interventions should be coupled with a stepped care approach for those requiring more targeted help.[49] Beyond an investment in school-based mental health, governments need to invest in the training of mental health care professionals. Indeed, far too many children and adolescents struggle with mental health challenges without adequate support—assessment waitlists are prohibitively long, as are treatment waitlists. The lower age thresholds that limit access to mental health care also need to be addressed. An intake age of 18 years for adult services is not supported by global metaepidemiological evidence and can deprive individuals of necessary care.[3]

SUMMARY AND DISCUSSION

Our review underscores the high prevalence of mental health challenges among children and adolescents prior to the pandemic, which has only escalated during and after the pandemic emergency.[29,31,33] The rates of impairment derived from clinical, epidemiologic, and developmental studies point to the fact that the mental health needs of children and adolescents were neither adequately prioritized before the pandemic nor during the pandemic.[18] The ongoing decline in child and adolescent mental health poses not only a significant risk at the individual level, but it also impacts economies and future generations. It is also true to say that existing evidence-based interventions for child and adolescent mental health are only moderately effective in reducing the burden of suffering associated with mental health challenges in this population. A clearer understanding of why there has been an increase in prevalence even prior to the pandemic is a crucial first step. There are many possible mechanisms including the financial crisis of 2008, the rapid and remarkable uptake of social media, and the increasing pressures on social institutions. Sophisticated research needs to be conducted that is developmentally and culturally sensitive to determine potential causal links between these societal influences and prevalence of mental disorders. This speaks to the need for population-based studies that are longitudinal in nature and that investigate both risk and protective factors in a dynamic interaction over time. Such research needs to be conducted especially in low and middle-income countries where most of the world's children and adolescents live.

CLINICS CARE POINTS

- Given the high prevalence of mental health disorder among children and adolescence, primary care providers and pediatricians need to be sensitive to the need for detection.
- Detection should occur over both childhood and adolescence as these 2 developmental periods are associated with variation in age of onset of mental disorders.
- There are certain subgroups of the population that are at higher risk of mental disorder than the general population. These include children and adolescents with physical health conditions, those living in poverty, and those affected by the social determinants of health, including racism.
- Universal and targeted interventions need to compliment clinical interventions to support all children and adolescents, as well as those at high risk and those with an already present clinical condition.
- Children and adolescents have less autonomy than adults and, as such, are more sensitive to their environment. Accordingly, the resilience of children and adolescents is contingent on the adults in the lives being healthy.[50] Addressing the family is thus key to helping children and adolescents.

DISCLOSURE

The authors have nothing to disclose.

REFERENCES

1. Kessler RC, Berglund P, Demler O, et al. Lifetime Prevalence and Age-of-Onset Distributions of DSM-IV Disorders in the National Comorbidity Survey Replication. Arch Gen Psychiatr 2005;62(6):593.
2. Kessler RC, Amminger GP, Aguilar-Gaxiola S, et al. Age of onset of mental disorders: a review of recent literature. Curr Opin Psychiatr 2007;20(4):359–64.
3. Solmi M, Radua J, Olivola M, et al. Age at onset of mental disorders worldwide: large-scale meta-analysis of 192 epidemiological studies. Mol Psychiatr 2022;27(1):281–95.
4. Polanczyk GV, Salum GA, Sugaya LS, et al. Annual Research Review: A meta-analysis of the worldwide prevalence of mental disorders in children and adolescents. JCPP (J Child Psychol Psychiatry) 2015;56(3):345–65.
5. Steinberg L. A social neuroscience perspective on adolescent risk-taking. Dev Rev 2008;28(1):78–106.
6. Crone EA, Dahl RE. Understanding adolescence as a period of social–affective engagement and goal flexibility. Nat Rev Neurosci 2012;13(9):636–50.
7. Kieling C, Buchweitz C, Caye A, et al. Worldwide Prevalence and Disability From Mental Disorders Across Childhood and Adolescence: Evidence From the Global Burden of Disease Study. JAMA Psychiatr 2024;31. https://doi.org/10.1001/jamapsychiatry.2023.5051.
8. Copeland WE, Wolke D, Shanahan L, et al. Adult Functional Outcomes of Common Childhood Psychiatric Problems: A Prospective, Longitudinal Study. JAMA Psychiatr 2015;72(9):892.
9. Erskine HE, Moffitt TE, Copeland WE, et al. A heavy burden on young minds: the global burden of mental and substance use disorders in children and youth. Psychol Med 2015;45(7):1551–63.

10. Krygsman A, Vaillancourt T. Elevated social anxiety symptoms across childhood and adolescence predict adult mental disorders and cannabis use. Compr Psychiatr 2022;115:152302.
11. Moitra M, Santomauro D, Degenhardt L, et al. Estimating the risk of suicide associated with mental disorders: A systematic review and meta-regression analysis. J Psychiatr Res 2021;137:242–9.
12. Cicchetti D, Rogosch FA. Equifinality and multifinality in developmental psychopathology. Dev Psychopathol 1996;8(4):597–600.
13. Page MJ, McKenzie JE, Bossuyt PM, et al. The PRISMA 2020 statement: an updated guideline for reporting systematic reviews. BMJ 2021;29:n71.
14. Brittain H, Vaillancourt T. Longitudinal associations between academic achievement and depressive symptoms in adolescence: Methodological considerations and analytical approaches for identifying temporal priority. Adv Child Dev Behav 2023;64:327–55. Elsevier.
15. Vaillancourt T, Brittain HL, McDougall P, et al. Longitudinal Links Between Childhood Peer Victimization, Internalizing and Externalizing Problems, and Academic Functioning: Developmental Cascades. J Abnorm Child Psychol 2013;41(8): 1203–15.
16. Curran PJ, Howard AL, Bainter SA, et al. The separation of between-person and within-person components of individual change over time: A latent curve model with structured residuals. J Consult Clin Psychol 2014;82(5):879–94.
17. Lee KS, Vaillancourt T. The role of childhood generalized anxiety in the internalizing cluster. Psychol Med 2020;50(13):2272–82.
18. Vaillancourt T, Szatmari P. Child Development, Major Disruptive Events—Public Health Implications. In: Oxford research encyclopedia of global public health. Oxford University Press; 2022. https://doi.org/10.1093/acrefore/9780190632366.013.159.
19. Vaillancourt T, Brittain H, Krygsman A, et al. Assessing the quality of research examining change in children's mental health in the context of COVID-19. Univ Ott J Med 2021;11(1). https://doi.org/10.18192/uojm.v11i1.5950.
20. Elia J, Pajer K, Prasad R, et al. Electronic health records identify timely trends in childhood mental health conditions. Child Adolesc Psychiatr Ment Health 2023; 17(1):107.
21. McGrath JJ, Al-Hamzawi A, Alonso J, et al. Age of onset and cumulative risk of mental disorders: a cross-national analysis of population surveys from 29 countries. Lancet Psychiatr 2023;10(9):668–81.
22. Reiss F. Socioeconomic inequalities and mental health problems in children and adolescents: A systematic review. Soc Sci Med 2013;90:24–31.
23. DuPont-Reyes MJ, Villatoro AP. The role of school race/ethnic composition in mental health outcomes: A systematic literature review. J Adolesc 2019;74(1): 71–82.
24. Lu W, Todhunter-Reid A, Mitsdarffer ML, et al. Barriers and Facilitators for Mental Health Service Use Among Racial/Ethnic Minority Adolescents: A Systematic Review of Literature. Front Public Health 2021;9:641605.
25. Williams AJ, Jones C, Arcelus J, et al. A systematic review and meta-analysis of victimisation and mental health prevalence among LGBTQ+ young people with experiences of self-harm and suicide. In: De Luca V, editor. PLoS One 2021; 16(1):e0245268.
26. Romano I, Buchan C, Baiocco-Romano L, et al. Physical-mental multimorbidity in children and youth: a scoping review. BMJ Open 2021;11(5):e043124.

27. Racine N, McArthur BA, Cooke JE, et al. Global Prevalence of Depressive and Anxiety Symptoms in Children and Adolescents During COVID-19: A Meta-analysis. JAMA Pediatr 2021;175(11):1142.
28. Alizadeh S, Shahrousvand S, Sepandi M, et al. Prevalence of anxiety, depression and post-traumatic stress disorder symptoms in children and adolescents during the COVID-19 pandemic: A systematic review and meta-analysis. J Public Health 2023. https://doi.org/10.1007/s10389-023-02168-w.
29. Madigan S, Racine N, Vaillancourt T, et al. Changes in Depression and Anxiety Among Children and Adolescents From Before to During the COVID-19 Pandemic: A Systematic Review and Meta-analysis. JAMA Pediatr 2023; 177(6):567.
30. Farrell AH, Vitoroulis I, Eriksson M, et al. Loneliness and Well-Being in Children and Adolescents during the COVID-19 Pandemic: A Systematic Review. Children 2023;10(2):279.
31. Madigan S, Korczak DJ, Vaillancourt T, et al. Comparison of paediatric emergency department visits for attempted suicide, self-harm, and suicidal ideation before and during the COVID-19 pandemic: a systematic review and meta-analysis. Lancet Psychiatr 2023;10(5):342–51.
32. Levine DA, Oh PS, Nash KA, et al. Pediatric Mental Health Emergencies During 5 COVID-19 Waves in New York City. Pediatrics 2023;152(5). e2022060553.
33. Madigan S, Vaillancourt T, Dimitropoulos G, et al. A Systematic Review and Meta-Analysis: Child and Adolescent Healthcare Utilization for Eating Disorders During the COVID-19 Pandemic. J Am Acad Child Adolesc Psychiatry 2024. https://doi.org/10.1016/j.jaac.2024.02.009. S0890856724000777.
34. Rogers MA, MacLean J. ADHD Symptoms Increased During the Covid-19 Pandemic: A Meta-Analysis. J Atten Disord 2023;27(8):800–11.
35. Antoniou T, Pajer K, Gardner W, et al. Impact of COVID-19 pandemic on prescription stimulant use among children and youth: a population-based study. Eur Child Adolesc Psychiatr 2024. https://doi.org/10.1007/s00787-023-02346-x.
36. Layman HM, Thorisdottir IE, Halldorsdottir T, et al. Substance Use Among Youth During the COVID-19 Pandemic: a Systematic Review. Curr Psychiatr Rep 2022; 24(6):307–24.
37. Centers for Disease Control and Prevention. CDC WONDER database. 2020. Available at: https://wonder.cdc.gov/.
38. Friedman J, Hadland SE. The Overdose Crisis among U.S. Adolescents. N Engl J Med 2024;390(2):97–100.
39. Friedman J, Godvin M, Shover CL, et al. Trends in Drug Overdose Deaths Among US Adolescents, January 2010 to June 2021. JAMA 2022;327(14):1398.
40. Hawke LD, Szatmari P, Cleverley K, et al. Youth in a pandemic: a longitudinal examination of youth mental health and substance use concerns during COVID-19. BMJ Open 2021;11(10):e049209.
41. Vaillancourt T, Farrell AH, Brittain H, et al. Bullying before and during the COVID-19 pandemic. Curr Opin Psychol 2023;53:101689.
42. McDougall P, Vaillancourt T. Long-term adult outcomes of peer victimization in childhood and adolescence: Pathways to adjustment and maladjustment. Am Psychol 2015;70(4):300–10.
43. Moore SE, Norman RE, Suetani S, et al. Consequences of bullying victimization in childhood and adolescence: A systematic review and meta-analysis. World J Psychiatr 2017;7(1):60.

44. Durbin A, Moineddin R, Lin E, et al. Mental health service use by recent immigrants from different world regions and by non-immigrants in Ontario, Canada: a cross-sectional study. BMC Health Serv Res 2015;15(1):336.
45. Merikangas KR, He JP, Burstein M, et al. Service Utilization for Lifetime Mental Disorders in U.S. Adolescents: Results of the National Comorbidity Survey–Adolescent Supplement (NCS-A). J Am Acad Child Adolesc Psychiatry 2011;50(1):32–45.
46. Georgiades K, Duncan L, Wang L, et al, 2014 Ontario Child Health Study Team. 2014 Ontario Child Health Study Team. Six-Month Prevalence of Mental Disorders and Service Contacts among Children and Youth in Ontario: Evidence from the 2014 Ontario Child Health Study. Can J Psychiatr 2019;64(4):246–55.
47. UNESCO. Global monitoring of school closures. 2024. Available at: https://covid19.uis.unesco.org/global-monitoring-school-closures-covid19/.
48. Vaillancourt T, Szatmari P, Georgiades K, et al. The impact of COVID-19 on the mental health of Canadian children and youth. Blais JM. FACETS 2021;6:1628–48.
49. Salloum A, Wang W, Robst J, et al. Stepped care versus standard trauma-focused cognitive behavioral therapy for young children. JCPP (J Child Psychol Psychiatry) 2016;57(5):614–22.
50. Vaillancourt T, Luthar SS. Stop assuming most kids will be resilient in the face of COVID-19: When we believe this, we fail to protect them as we must. 2022. Available at: https://rsc-src.ca/en/voices/stop-assuming-most-kids-will-be-resilient-in-face-covid-19-when-we-believe-this-we-fail-to.

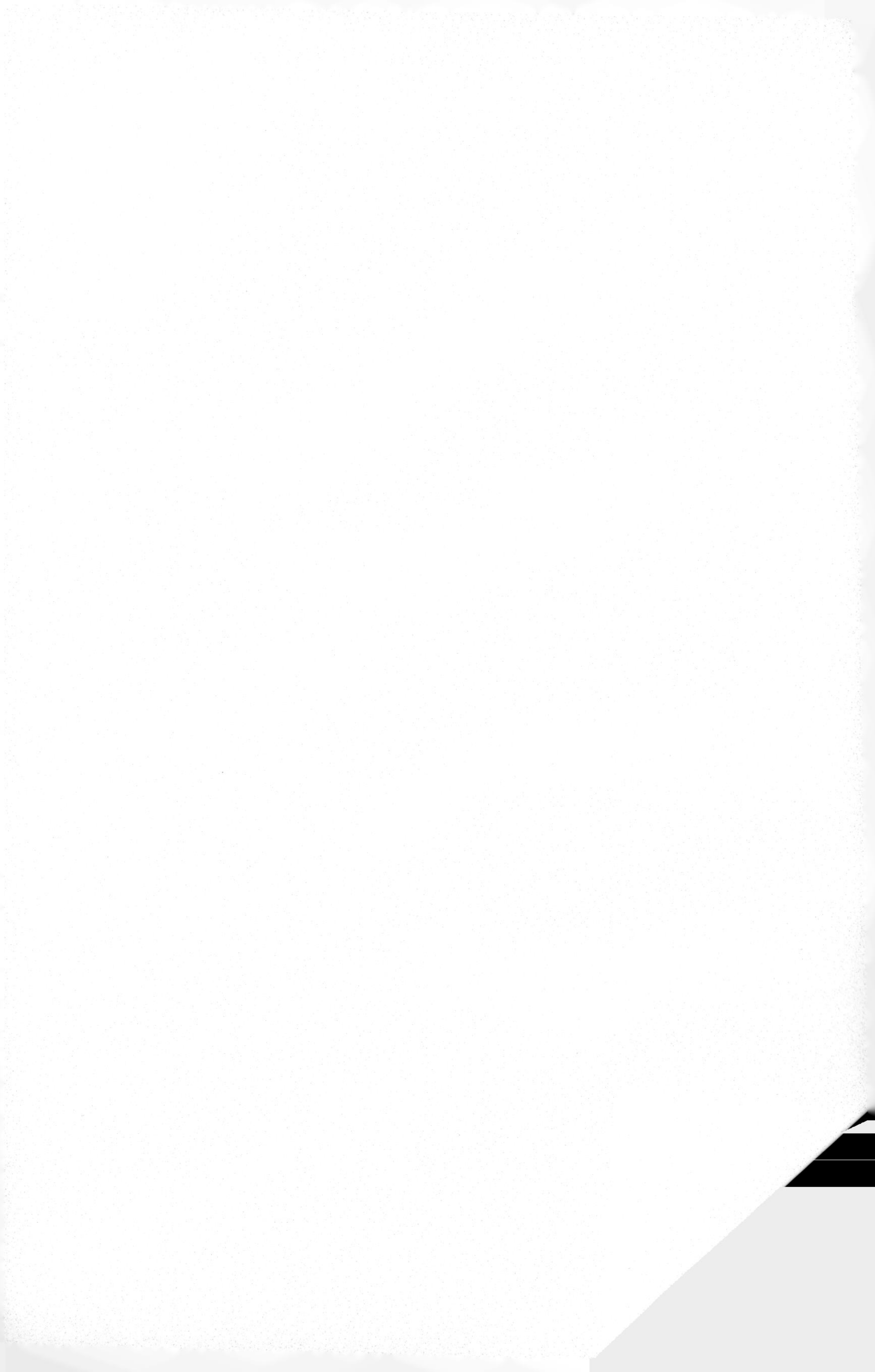

Mental Health Screening and Measurement in Children and Adolescents

Marie Reilly, MD*, Carol Weitzman, MD

KEYWORDS

• Pediatric • Mental and behavioral health • Screening • Suicide • Depression • Anxiety

KEY POINTS

- The United States is facing a pediatric behavioral and mental health crisis with approximately 20% of children experiencing a mental, emotional, or behavioral health problem each year and 40% meeting criteria for a disorder by the age of 18 years.
- The American Academy of Pediatrics recommends that global and domain-specific screening for mental, emotional, and behavioral concerns begin early in a child's life and occur at every routine health maintenance visit.
- Screening should be embedded within a broader system of ongoing, regular surveillance in primary care that promotes longitudinal relationships with children and families, identifies family and child strengths, and explores concerns and child and family needs.

BACKGROUND

The United States is currently facing a pediatric behavioral and mental health crisis. An estimated 20% of children aged 17 years or under experience a mental, emotional, or behavioral health problem each year and 40% will meet criteria for a disorder by the age of 18 years.[1] The most prevalent disorders include attention deficit/hyperactivity disorder (ADHD) and anxiety with each affecting nearly 10% of children. Approximately 20% of adolescents experienced a major depressive episode and approximately 17% of children aged between 2 and 8 years are diagnosed with mental health, emotional, developmental, or/and behavioral problems.[2] The high rates of mental, emotional, and behavioral health problems predated the coronavirus disease 2019 (COVID-19) pandemic,[1,3] but rates further increased in the setting of the COVID-19 pandemic with nearly 1 in 6 children reporting symptoms of anxiety or depression.[4] Similarly, suicide rates among youth began to climb long before the pandemic and

Division of Developmental Medicine, Boston Children's Hospital, 300 Longwood Avenue, BCH 3217, Boston, MA 02115, USA
* Corresponding author.
E-mail address: Marie.reilly@childrens.harvard.edu

Pediatr Clin N Am 71 (2024) 1013–1026
https://doi.org/10.1016/j.pcl.2024.07.010 **pediatric.theclinics.com**

sharply increased by 56% between 2007 and 2017 for persons aged 10 to 24 years. Suicide is now the second leading cause of death in the United States among those aged 10 to 24 years.[5] In addition, children and adolescents with mental health concerns frequently face unmet needs as well as prolonged time to intervention.[6]

Between 2013 and 2019, approximately 10% of youth aged between 3 and 17 years as well as 25% of youth aged 12 to 17 years received mental health services. Up to 7.8% of youth aged 13 to 17 years report taking medication for a mental health, emotional, or behavioral issue.[3] Despite the alarmingly high prevalence and even treatment rates, there continues to be an underidentification and treatment of youth.

Given that primary pediatric care is characterized frequent visits, longitudinal care, and a focus on prevention, primary care clinicians are well positioned to both identify mental, emotional, and behavioral health concerns and initiate intervention.[7] In fact, not only are they well positioned but also they can be considered the country's "de facto mental health system."[8]

BARRIERS TO SCREENING

Although rates of routine mental health screening are higher among urban primary care practices, screening is far from universal.[6,9] Primary care clinicians often receive limited training in the assessment of mental or behavioral health concerns or in implementation of evidence-based interventions during their training.[8,10] In the example of suicide screening, identified barriers to screening include clinicians'

- Limited knowledge of suicide risk
- Personal discomfort
- Time constraints
- Electronic medical record limitations, and
- Lack of an adequate tool.[9]

Clinicians may also be unsure as to how to interpret a positive mental health screen or how to explain the meaning of the results to the patient or their caregivers.[6,11] Surveyed pediatricians have reported a lack of training and confidence in treating children with mental, emotional, and behavior problems as a barrier to screening.[12] In surveys administered in 2004 and 2013, however, pediatricians were less likely to report inadequate training in identifying concerns, time, and reimbursement as a barrier to screening in 2013.[12]

CURRENT STATE OF DETECTION OF MENTAL HEALTH, EMOTIONAL, AND BEHAVIORAL CONCERNS

Research indicates that many children and adolescents with significant mental, emotional, or behavioral concerns are not routinely detected in the primary care setting. Standardized screening tools significantly improve the primary care provider's ability to identify these areas of concern as clinical judgment alone, in the absence of a screening tool results in a sensitivity of 14% to 54% and a specificity of 69% to 100% to detect problems.[13] Screening addresses an equity issue as primary care clinicians are, otherwise, less likely to identify mental, emotional, or behavioral health concerns in children of color and in non-English-speaking patients.[14] Screening can reduce implicit biases that may lead to underdiagnosis or misdiagnosis. When children with mental, emotional, or behavioral concerns are identified, they are more likely to receive treatment.[15]

In comparison with rates of developmental screening in primary care, there is limited research on screening for mental, emotional, and behavior problems. A number of promising new strategies have been introduced to improve screening rates such as American Academy of Pediatrics (AAP) Extension for Community Healthcare Outcomes trainings, learning collaboratives, and integration of mental health clinicians into pediatric practices.[16–18] With these types of interventions, screening rates have been shown to improve dramatically, increasing from 1% before the initiative to 74% afterward.[16]

STANDARDIZED SCREENING MEASURES

Screening should not occur in isolation and should be embedded within a broader system of ongoing, regular surveillance in primary care. Whereas surveillance is "a flexible, longitudinal, and continuous process whereby knowledgeable professionals perform skilled observations during the provision of health care," screening is a procedure that is notable for the use of standardized tools.[19] Both screening and surveillance present an opportunity to initiate conversations with children and families, explore concerns, identify caregiver and child strengths, and discuss the significance of findings that may be detected on a screen.

Successful screening depends on several factors associated with the standardized measure including the sensitivity and specificity as well as the positive and negative predictive value. Sensitivity refers to the ability to detect those who have a condition (rule-in).[20] Specificity is the ability to detect those who do not have a condition (rule-out[20]; **Table 1**). The positive predictive value of a screen is the probability that a youth with a positive screen actually have the condition for which they are being screened.[21] The negative predictive value is the probability that a youth with negative screen does not have the condition for which they are being screened.[21] Primary care clinicians need to be aware of the sociodemographic characteristics of the normative population used to validate a measure to ensure that the screening measure chosen reflects the population for whom it is being used. There is currently no consensus on the appropriate values of sensitivity and specificity for these type of screening measures.[22]

No single measure is appropriate for children of all ages. General or global screening measures evaluate multiple areas of mental, emotional, and behavioral functioning while domain-specific screens evaluate one area of functioning (eg, ADHD, depression or anxiety). A list of mental, emotional, and behavioral screens that are found in the public domain are listed in **Table 2**. A more comprehensive list of mental health screening measures can be accessed through the Mental Health Initiatives webpage of the AAP.[23]

Child self-report versions exist for several screening measures and are important to include, as children may not always disclose their feelings or state of mind to their caregivers. Many screens are available for children aged over 8 years, and the cognitive and literacy level of the child will influence when these are used. Teacher reports can also augment caregiver and self-report and provide insight into a child's functioning in school.

Table 1
Screening measure assessment

	Sensitivity	Specificity
Definition	The ability to detect those who have a condition	The ability to detect those who do not have a condition
Mnemonic	SPIN: SPecific tests rule IN the condition when they are positive	SNOUT: SeNsitive tests rule OUT the condition when they are negative

Table 2
Commonly available mental health, emotional, and behavioral screening tools

Measure Name	Ages	Number of Items	Informants
General Behavioral Screening			
SWYC (The Survey of Well-Being of Young Children): Baby Pediatric Symptom Checklist	1–18 mo	12	Caregiver
ASQ:SE 2 (Ages and Stages Questionnaire: Social Emotional 2)	1–72 mo	9 age-specific forms with 19–33 items	Caregiver
SWYC (The Survey of Well-Being of Young Children): Preschool Pediatric Symptom Checklist	18–65 mo	18	Caregiver
SDQ (Strengths and Difficulties Questionnaire)	2–17 y	25	Child, caregivers, or teacher
PSC-17b (Pediatric Symptom Checklist-17)	4–18 y	17	Caregiver
PSC-17Y	11+ y	17	Child
PSC-35	11+ y	35	Caregiver
Anxiety			
Spence Children's Anxiety Scale	Caregiver-completed for ages 2.5–6.5 y Child-completed for ages 8–12 y	Child: 34–45 Caregiver: 35–45	Child and caregiver
SCARED (Self-Report for Child Anxiety Related Emotional Disorders)	8+ y	41	Child and caregivers
GAD-7 (Generalized Anxiety Disorder-7)	12+ y	7	Child
Depression			
PHQ-2 (Patient Health Questionnaire-2)	12+ y	2	Child
PHQ-9 (Patient Health Questionnaire-9)	12+ y	9 plus severity items	Child

Suicide			
Adapted-SAD PERSONS	Elementary and middle school-age	10	Child
ASQ (Ask Suicide-Screening Questions)	8+ y	4	Child
CSSR (Columbia Suicide Severity Rating Scale)	11+ y	6+	Child
PHQ-A (Patient Health Questionnaire for Adolescents)	13–18 y	11	Child
ADHD			
ADHD Rating Scale-5	5–17 y	18	Caregiver and teacher
Vanderbilt Diagnostic Rating Scale	6–12 y	Caregiver: 55 items Teacher: 43 items	Caregivers and teachers
Maternal Depression			
Edinburgh Postnatal Depression Scale	18+ years	10	Caregiver

The Ages and Stages Questionnaire has an initial cost, but materials can be photocopied.

Emerging data suggest that in the era of telemedicine, screening may be less likely to happen.[24] Families with higher social determinants of health (SDOHs) and less social support are more likely to miss routine health maintenance visits.[25] For these reasons, clinicians need to consider screening children at other encounters within the pediatric practice, such as during acute care visits.[26]

Some mental, emotional, and behavioral health screening measures can be administered through a patient portal within the electronic health record (EHR) and incorporated into the medical record, facilitating documentation of screening and tracking screening rates.[27] However, this is not possible across all measures often due to copyright issues. Private software systems have emerged to fill this gap by offering primary care practices a suite of supports including previsit questionnaires, patient health education, patient tracking, and clinical note facilitation.[28] In the future, mental health screening initiatives may expand beyond the primary care setting. Specifically, the Patient Health Questionnaire-9 (PHQ-9) has recently been explored for its potential for use in broader community settings like pharmacies and schools in order to identify more children with problems and provide greater access to mental health care.[11] Work will need to be done to ensure that these screens are incorporated into the medical record and that primary care clinicians are aware of these findings.

UPDATES TO MENTAL AND BEHAVIORAL HEALTH SCREENING GUIDELINES

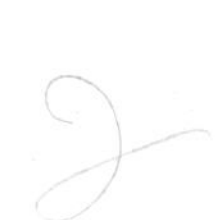

- In 2016, the US Preventative Services Task Force (USPSTF) recommended routine screening for depression in children and adolescents (aged 12–18 years) in the primary care setting but did not find sufficient evidence to recommend screening in children aged 11 years or under.[17]
- In 2022, the USPSTF affirmed the recommendation earlier.[29] The Guidelines for Adolescent Depression in Primary Care (GLAD-PC) also recommended annual screening for depression in children and adolescents aged older than 12 years.[17] However, in addition to annual screening, GLAD-PC also recommended more frequent screening for depression during health care encounters for individuals aged 10 to 21 years who have additional risk factors for depression due to the increased likelihood of developing depression in the future.[30] These risk factors for depression in the adolescent population include a history of previous depressive episodes, positive family history, the presence of other mental, emotional, and behavioral conditions, substance use, trauma exposure, psychosocial stressors, somatic complaints, and previously elevated depression screens that did not meet criteria for a depression diagnosis.[30]
- In 2022, the USPSTF recommended annual screening for anxiety in youth aged 8 to 18 years.[31]
- They also reported that there was insufficient evidence to recommend screening for suicide risk in children and adolescents.[31] In response to this, the AAP, the American Foundation for Suicide Prevention, and National Institute of Mental Health (NIMH) released the "Blueprint for Youth Suicide Prevention" recommending annual universal screening for suicide risk in youth aged 12 years or older and as clinically indicated for children aged 8 to 11 years.[32]

As a result of these recommendations and the growing mental health crisis in children, in 2022, the AAP updated the Bright Futures Recommendations for Preventive Pediatric Health Care to reflect a shift in the primary care model such that while clinicians should continue to engage in longitudinal psychosocial and behavioral surveillance at every health supervision visit, mental, emotional, and behavioral health screening should also be completed at every routine health maintenance visit.[33] The recent changes to AAP recommendations outline the need for clinicians to utilize both screening and surveillance in order to best support their patients and to maximize the likelihood of detecting mental, emotional, and behavioral health problems.

CURRENT SCREENING RECOMMENDATIONS

Current recommended mental, emotional, and behavioral screening intervals are shown in **Table 3**. Screening should begin in the first year of life as recent studies have shown that not only can problems be detected in young children but also many children will have elevated levels of symptom severity that present early in life.[7] As these problems have a high likelihood of persistence, beginning screening early in life, when problems can be ameliorated, is critical. Pediatric clinicians need to select screening tools that are feasible and appropriate for their practice. The length of time required to complete and score them as well as their availability in multiple languages are important considerations. Reported sensitivity and specificity often have a wide range, reflecting the various populations and settings where screens have been administered. These ranges also reinforce that screening results are most effectively used to initiate conversations with children and caregivers.

General Mental, Emotional, and Behavioral Concerns

Global screening measures evaluate multiple domains of mental, emotional, and behavioral functioning and 2 of the most commonly used screens in pediatric primary care include the Pediatric Symptom Checklist (PSC) and the Strengths and Difficulties Questionnaire (SDQ; see **Table 2**). These measures have been found to have a sensitivity ranging from 63% to 95% with a specificity of 68% to 98%. In a large sample of caregiver completed screens, the 17 item PSC identified 11.6% of children with positive screens, which was fairly evenly distributed between internalizing and externalizing disorders.[34] Global screening has been shown to detect adolescent depression reasonably well, although the addition of a domain-specific depression measure helps identify additional youth that global screening does not capture.[35] Global measures have also been shown to be a useful adjunct to suicide screening by helping to assess clinical severity and the range of other psychosocial problems.[36] If a global screen is positive, primary care clinicians can consider administering a more domain-specific screen, such as an ADHD measure.

Anxiety and Depression

Two commonly used screens for anxiety include the Screen for Child Anxiety Related Disorders (SCARED) and the Generalized Anxiety Disorder-7 (GAD-7) scale. The sensitivity and specificity of the SCARED range from 50% to 88% and 56% to 98%, respectively.[37,38] There are a number of commonly used depression screens including the PHQ series. The PHQ-2 is a brief 2 question depression screen that asks about the patient's experience of having "little interest or pleasure in doing things" or "feeling down, depressed, or hopeless" in the past 2 weeks. A score greater or equal to 3 has been associated with a sensitivity of 74% to 87% and a specificity of 75% to 92% for detecting major depression in a primary care setting.[39]

Suicide

Suicide screening has more recently emerged as an area for potential intervention within primary care due to the rising rates. In addition to rising rates of completed suicides, rates of suicidal ideation and suicide attempts have also been increasing.[40] Many youths seek health care of some kind within a month of attempting suicide.[9]

Table 3
Recommended screening intervals

Mental, Emotional, and Behavioral Screening Recommendations			
Age	**Interval**	**Screening Recommendations**	**Screen Completer**
Birth to 6 mo	Each health maintenance visit	• Maternal depression • Global screen	Caregiver
7 mo to 7 y	Yearly	• Global screen • Consider anxiety screen if indicated	Caregiver
8–11 y	Yearly	• Global screen • Anxiety screen • Consider depression and suicide screen if indicated	Caregiver Self-report if able
12 y and older	Yearly	• Global screen • Anxiety screen • Depression screen • Suicide screen	Caregiver Self-report if able

In the pediatric population, suicide risk screening can identify youth who were *not* detected on depression screens.[41] In fact, depression screening alone misses up to 25% of youth at risk of suicide.[9] The Ask Suicide-Screening Questions (ASQ) has been found to have a sensitivity of 96.7% and a specificity of 91.1% among hospitalized pediatric patients.[42] However, there is some concern that current suicide risk screening measures may not be applicable to broader pediatric populations or to children with neurodevelopmental disabilities.[43]

The PHQ-9 is a commonly utilized screening tool for depression in primary care given its psychometric validity, brevity, and availability, as well as its ability to be integrated into the medical record.[11,40] The American Academy of Child and Adolescent Psychiatry modified the PHQ-9 to the Patient Health Questionnaire for Adolescents (PHQ-A), which was validated for use among those aged 13 to 18 years.[37] The PHQ-A differs from the PHQ-9 in that it includes 2 questions related to suicide ("Has there been a time in the past month when you have had serious thoughts about ending your life?" and "Have you ever, in your whole life, tried to kill yourself or made a suicide attempt?"). The PHQ-A has been associated with a specificity of 84% to 95% and a sensitivity of 68% to 95% to detect suicidal ideation in a population of adolescent athletes.[44] Based on the responses to these questions, the primary care provider may consider using a second screener, like the ASQ, to improve sensitivity, which can take under a minute to administer.[40] If the patient responds affirmatively to any of the 4 questions, the clinician asks one additional acuity question.[45] The Joint Commission has approved the ASQ for use in all ages.[46]

RELATED SCREENS

Social Determinants of Health

SDOHs refer to the social circumstances in which individuals live and work.[47] Within pediatrics, examples of SDOHs include child maltreatment, childcare and education needs, finances, physical environment, caregiver social support, intimate partner violence, maternal depression and caregiver mental health, substance abuse, firearm exposure, and caregiver health literacy (Chung). There is a strong relationship between having mental, emotional, and behavior problems, such as anxiety and depression, posttraumatic stress disorder and suicidal ideation, and experiencing more adverse SDOHs.[48] Therefore, identifying SDOH challenges in a family should alert clinicians to a higher risk of mental, emotional, and behavioral health problems in a child, and vice versa. Having this information could provide opportunities to connect caregivers with necessary supports that may include psychosocial interventions beyond mental health counseling.

Maternal Depression

Screening for maternal depression plays an important role in screening for the well-being of children and families. While the parent is not under the care of the pediatric provider, pediatric clinicians may be better positioned to detect postpartum depression than obstetricians given the frequency of well-checks in the first year of life.[49] As a result, the AAP now recommends screening for maternal depression at the 1, 2, 4, and 6 months well visits (see **Table 3**).[33]

Trauma

Children living in poverty are at an increased risk of trauma. Children from families of low socioeconomic status experience a 5 times greater risk of abuse and neglect.[50] Given the elevated risk of trauma among children living in poverty, primary care clinicians may consider using domain-specific trauma screening in children experiencing adversity related to SDOHs who screen positive on mental, emotional, and behavioral screening measures.

DISCUSSING A POSITIVE SCREEN

A positive screen can indicate the detection of an underlying mental, emotional, or behavioral concern and may suggest the severity of impairment.

- Initially, a clinician needs to discuss the findings of the screen to gauge caregivers' and children's reactions to the findings and explore their concerns.
- Conditions like inadequate or poor-quality sleep, inadequate nutrition, limited exercise, environmental stressors, and excessive media use can negatively impact child functioning and result in a positive screen or exacerbate mental, emotional, or behavioral problems. It is important to query these areas to clarify the presence of these contributing factors.
- Primary care clinicians can consider utilizing communication techniques to help facilitate a therapeutic alliance.[51] The mnemonic HEL^{2}P^3 outlines a communication strategy in which the clinician offers hope, empathy, uses the caregiver's own language to describe the concern, expresses loyalty, asks permission to query further, partners with the family, and creates a plan.[51]
- The clinician needs to assess the impact of symptoms on the child's functioning at home, school, and in the community. Together with the caregivers and the child depending on their age, a plan, using shared decision-making, can be developed to initiate appropriate treatment and/or follow-up.
- The time to follow-up within primary care may differ depending on the degree of impairment the child is experiencing.

MANAGEMENT OF A POSITIVE SUICIDE SCREEN

Management of a positive suicide screen requires that the primary care provider take additional steps to assess severity of symptoms and appropriate disposition. Before a primary care provider screens for suicide, they must discuss the boundaries of confidentiality. Specifically, clinicians should emphasize that the content discussed between the primary care provider and adolescent will remain confidential except for information related to safety including self-harm, suicidality, or homicidality. When speaking with caregivers about suicidality, primary care clinicians should recognize that parents often have limited awareness of their child's thoughts about suicide.[40] In particular, fathers have demonstrated particular vulnerabilities in their awareness of their child's thoughts about suicide and death.[52] Parents from racial minorities are also less likely to be aware of their child's thoughts about suicide and death, with the exception being Hispanic parents who were more likely to know about their child's thoughts about death.[52]

If the child discloses suicidality or a suicide-screening tool is positive, the primary care provider's next step is to conduct a brief suicide safety assessment.[45] The NIMH recommends that a brief suicide safety assessment that includes praising the child for disclosing their thoughts, asking further questions about depressive symptoms, a suicide plan, past suicidal behavior, social supports and stressors, as well as assessing the frequency of suicidal thoughts.[45] After addressing these areas, a safety plan should be created in order to manage future suicidal thoughts.[45] Safety planning should also include counseling caregivers to remove access to means of completing suicide like medications and firearms.[40]

Based on the results of the brief suicide safety assessment, the provider must then decide on the child's disposition. If the child is determined to be at significant risk of suicide, they should go to the emergency room or other acute care setting for further evaluation.[45] If the child is not at imminent risk of suicide, then the provider should refer for further mental health support and maintain close follow-up.[45]

FUTURE DIRECTIONS

Current vulnerabilities in the screening process pertain to privacy during screen completion as well as how screening is explained and by whom in the practice.[6] Computerized screening may be able to address these areas and to facilitate efficient administration, scoring, tracking, and integration of results into the visit note within the EHR as well as decision-making support for the clinician.[6,53] Electronic platforms may also be able to address some current challenges related to screening including accessibility for individuals with sensory impairments or vulnerable health literacy, which are not currently feasible with paper screening measures.[6,22] However, additional research is needed as screens may perform differently depending on how they are administered.[54]

As the role of patient-generated health data and previsit questionnaires continues to grow in clinical settings, there may be greater opportunities to obtain adolescent self-reported concerns through novel technological platforms or applications.[55] Artificial intelligence (AI) and machine learning may also improve mental health screening in the future, particularly with respect to diagnostic support and treatment recommendations. Prediction models, generated by machine learning, are being utilized to create clinical decision support systems related to regarding risk assessment determination in individuals presenting to emergency departments due to self-harm.[56] However, at this time, AI is not capable of providing reliable support, with respect to diagnostics or recommendations, in the area of pediatric behavioral or mental health.[57] Given the importance of mental health screening and the need for timely, evidence-based intervention, there is a need for further innovation related to the goals of increasing the rates of pediatric mental health screening and of decreasing the time to evidence-based treatment.

CLINICS CARE POINTS

- Alarming rates of children have mental, emotional, and behavioral health problems necessitating a need for a broader means to identify children and help them obtain treatment.
- The AAP recommends that global and domain-specific screening for mental, emotional, and behavioral concerns begin early in a child's life and occur at every routine health maintenance visit.
- ... commendations, anxiety screening should begin after the age of ... nd suicide risk screening after the age of 12 years unless earlier ... icated.
- ... edded within a broader system of ongoing, regular surveillance in ... nd surveillance present an opportunity to develop longitudinal ... and families and to identify family and child strengths, initiate ... concerns and needs.
- ... sures in primary care should be selected based on their feasibility ... ormative population in whom they were tested should reflect the ... being used.

- Screening results should trigger a conversation with caregivers and children to explore findings and determine next best steps.
- Children who screen positive for suicide must be assessed for the risk of imminent harm with an appropriate action plan put in place.

DISCLOSURE

The authors have no commercial or financial conflicts of interest.

REFERENCES

1. Shim R, Szilagyi M, Perrin JM. Epidemic rates of child and adolescent mental health disorders require an urgent response. Pediatrics 2022;149(5). https://doi.org/10.1542/peds.2022-056611.
2. Data and Statistics on Children's Mental Health. Centers for Disease Control and Prevention, National Center for Injury Prevention and Control.
3. Bitsko RH, Claussen AH, Lichstein J, et al. Mental health surveillance among children - United States, 2013-2019. MMWR Suppl 2022;71(2):1–42.
4. Zablotsky B, Black LI, Terlizzi EP, et al. Anxiety and depression symptoms among children before and during the COVID-19 pandemic. Ann Epidemiol 2022;75:53–6.
5. Curtin SC, Heron M. Death Rates Due to Suicide and Homicide Among Persons Aged 10–24: United States, 2000–2017. National Center for Health Statistics, Division of Vital Statistics.
6. Wissow LS, Brown J, Fothergill KE, et al. Universal mental health screening in pediatric primary care: a systematic review. J Am Acad Child Adolesc Psychiatry 2013;52(11):1134–47.e23.
7. Ammerman RT, Mara CA, Anyigbo C, et al. Behavior problems in low-income young children screened in pediatric primary care. JAMA Pediatr 2023;177(12):1306–13.
8. Petts RA, Gaynor ST. Behavioral health in primary care: brief screening and intervention strategies for pediatric clinicians. Pediatr Clin North Am 2021;68(3):583–606.
9. Milliman CC, Dwyer PA, Vessey JA. Pediatric suicide screening: a review of the evidence. J Pediatr Nurs 2021;59:1–9.
10. Horowitz L, Tipton MV, Pao M. Primary and secondary prevention of youth suicide. Pediatrics 2020;145(Suppl 2):S195–203.
11. Costantini L, Pasquarella C, Odone A, et al. Screening for depression in primary care with Patient Health Questionnaire-9 (PHQ-9): a systematic review. J Affect Disord 2021;279:473–83.
12. Horwitz SM, Storfer-Isser A, Kerker BD, et al. Barriers to the identification and management of psychosocial problems: changes from 2004 to 2013. Acad Pediatr 2015;15(6):613–20.
13. Sheldrick RC, Merchant S, Perrin EC. Identification of developmental-behavioral problems in primary care: a systematic review. Pediatrics 2011;128(2):356–63.
14. Gardner W, Kelleher KJ, Pajer KA, et al. Primary care clinicians' use of standardize tools to assess child psychosocial problems. Ambul Pediatr 2003;3(4):191–5.
15. Ghandour RM, Sherman LJ, Vladutiu CJ, et al. Prevalence and treatment of d sion, anxiety, and conduct problems in US children. J Pediatr 2019;206:2
16. Beers LS, Godoy L, John T, et al. Mental health screening quality i learning collaborative in pediatric primary care. Pediatrics 2017 doi.org/10.1542/peds.2016-2966.

17. Beck A, LeBlanc JC, Morissette K, et al. Screening for depression in children and adolescents: a protocol for a systematic review update. Syst Rev 2021;10(1):24.
18. Harder VS, Barry SE, French S, et al. Improving adolescent depression screening in pediatric primary care. Acad Pediatr 2019;19(8):925–33.
19. Dworkin PH. British and American recommendations for developmental monitoring: the role of surveillance. Pediatrics 1989;84(6):1000–10.
20. Mental Health Screening and Assessment Tools for Primary Care. American Academy of Pediatrics.
21. Disease Screening - Statistics Teaching Tools. New York State Department of Health.
22. Weitzman C, Wegner L, Section on Developmental and Behavioral Pediatrics, et al. Promoting optimal development: screening for behavioral and emotional problems. Pediatrics 2015;135(2):384–95.
23. Mental Health Initiatives. American Academy of Pediatrics.
24. Blackstone SR, Sebring AN, Allen C, et al. Improving depression screening in primary care: a quality improvement initiative. J Community Health 2022;47(3):400–7.
25. Wolf ER, Hochheimer CJ, Sabo RT, et al. Gaps in well-child care attendance among primary care clinics serving low-income families. Pediatrics 2018; 142(5). https://doi.org/10.1542/peds.2017-4019.
26. Esposito J. Suicide screening and behavioral health assessment in the emergency departmENT. Clin Pediatr Emerg Med 2019;20(1):63–70.
27. Children's Electronic Health Record Format. Agency for Healthcare Research and Quality.
28. CHADIS. CHADIS Incorporated.
29. Final Recommendation Statement Depression and Suicide Risk in Children and Adolescents: Screening. U.S. Preventive Services Taskforce.
30. Zuckerbrot RA, Cheung A, Jensen PS, et al, GLAD-PC Steering Group. Guidelines for Adolescent Depression in Primary Care (GLAD-PC): Part I. Practice Preparation, identification, assessment, and initial management. Pediatrics 2018;141(3). https://doi.org/10.1542/peds.2017-4081.
31. Final Recommendation Ctatement Anxiety in Children and Adolescents: Screening. United States Preventive Services Task Force.
32. Suicide: Blueprint for Youth Suicide Prevention. American Academy of Pediatrics.
33. About Bright Futures. American Academy of Pediatrics.
34. Murphy JM, Bergmann P, Chiang C, et al. The PSC-17: subscale scores, reliability, and factor structure in a new national sample. Pediatrics 2016;138(3). https://doi.org/10.1542/peds.2016-0038.
35. Jellinek M, Bergmann P, Holcomb JM, et al. Recognizing adolescent depression with parent- and youth-report screens in pediatric primary care. J Pediatr 2021; 233:220–6.e1.
36. Holcomb JM, Dutta A, Bergmann P, et al. Suicidal ideation in adolescents: understanding results from screening with the PHQ-9M and the PSC-17P. J Dev Behav Pediatr 2022;43(6):346–52.
37. Johnson JG, Harris ES, Spitzer RL, et al. The patient health questionnaire for adolescents: validation of an instrument for the assessment of mental disorders among adolescent primary care patients. J Adolesc Health 2002;30(3):196–204.
38. Muris P, Merckelbach H, Kindt M, et al. The utility of Screen for Child Anxiety Related Emotional Disorders (SCARED) as a tool for identifying children at high risk for prevalent anxiety disorders. Hist Philos Logic: Int J 2001;14(3):265–83.

39. Richardson LP, Rockhill C, Russo JE, et al. Evaluation of the PHQ-2 as a brief screen for detecting major depression among adolescents. Pediatrics 2010; 125(5):e1097–103.
40. Breslin K, Balaban J, Shubkin CD. Adolescent suicide: what can pediatricians do? Curr Opin Pediatr 2020;32(4):595–600.
41. Kemper AR, Hostutler CA, Beck K, et al. Depression and suicide-risk screening results in pediatric primary care. Pediatrics 2021;148(1). https://doi.org/10.1542/peds.2021-049999.
42. Horowitz LM, Wharff EA, Mournet AM, et al. Validation and feasibility of the ASQ among pediatric medical and surgical inpatients. Hosp Pediatr 2020;10(9):750–7.
43. Ludi E, Ballard ED, Greenbaum R, et al. Suicide risk in youth with intellectual disabilities: the challenges of screening. J Dev Behav Pediatr 2012;33(5):431–40.
44. Long A, DeFreese JD, Bickett A, et al. Factorial validity and invariance of an adolescent depression symptom screening tool. J Athl Train 2022;57(6):592–8.
45. Ask Suicide-Screening Questions (ASQ) Toolkit. National Institute of Mental Health.
46. Suicide Prevention Resources to support Joint Commission Accredited organizations implementation of NPSG 15.01.01. The Joint Commission.
47. Chung EK, Siegel BS, Garg A, et al. Screening for social determinants of health among children and families living in poverty: a guide for clinicians. Curr Probl Pediatr Adolesc Health Care 2016;46(5):135–53.
48. Prokosch C, Fertig AR, Ojebuoboh AR, et al. Exploring associations between social determinants of health and mental health outcomes in families from socioeconomically and racially and ethnically diverse households. Prev Med 2022;161:107150.
49. Barkin JL, Van Cleve S. Screening for maternal mental health in the pediatric setting: situational stressors and supports. J Pediatr Health Care 2020;34(5):405–6.
50. Fast Facts: Preventing Child Abuse & Neglect. Centers for Disease Control and Prevention.
51. Common Factors Approach: HEL2P 3 to Build a Better Alliance. American Academy of Pediatrics.
52. Jones JD, Boyd RC, Calkins ME, et al. Parent-adolescent agreement about adolescents' suicidal thoughts. Pediatrics 2019;143(2). https://doi.org/10.1542/peds.2018-1771.
53. Beck KE, Snyder D, Toth C, et al. Improving primary care adolescent depression screening and initial management: a quality improvement study. Pediatr Qual Saf 2022;7(2):e549.
54. Patalay P, Hayes D, Deighton J, et al. A comparison of paper and computer administered strengths and difficulties questionnaire. J Psychopathol Behav Assess 2016;38(2):242–50.
55. Grout RW, Cheng ER, Aalsma MC, et al. Let them speak for themselves: improving adolescent self-report rate on pre-visit screening. Acad Pediatr 2019;19(5):581–8.
56. Mortier P, Amigo F, Bhargav M, et al. Developing a clinical decision support system software prototype that assists in the management of patients with self-harm in the emergency department: protocol of the PERMANENS project. BMC Psychiatry 2024;24(1):220.
57. Kim R, Margolis A, Barile J, et al. Challenging the Chatbot: an assessment of chatGPT's diagnoses and recommendations for DBP case studies. J Dev Behav Pediatr 2024;45(1):e8–13.

Relational Health in Pediatrics

David W. Willis, MD[a,*], Dayna Long, MD[b], Kay Johnson, MPH, EdM[c]

KEYWORDS

• Child health care • Early relational health • Maternal child health
• Parent-child interactions • Equity • Pediatrics

KEY POINTS

- The concept of flourishing has been well-documented and defined in adults, but less has been known about flourishing and its correlates among children.
- The American Academy of Pediatrics 2021 Policy Statement called for a paradigm shift that would prioritize clinical activities, rewrite research agendas, and realign collective advocacy by promoting relational health in partnership with communities and families.
- Parent-child interactions are known to have impact on later mental and social well-being.
- Despite the documented advantages of having a medical home and its promotion by governmental, professional, and family advocacy organizations, too few United States' children have a medical home.

OVERVIEW

The paradigm shift toward early relational health (ERH) has emerged in child health care, public health, and early childhood system building as a major transformational catalyst to advance innovations for child heath practice, research, and policy.[1–7] ERH is defined as the state of emotional well-being that grows from the positive emotional connection that babies and toddlers and their parents/caregivers experience with each other through every day moments of caregiving and nurturing.[8] This relational framework builds upon decades of brain science, human development, and infant mental health research and focuses on the critical early relational experiences that are now understood as key drivers for child development, lifelong health, and flourishing.[1,9–13] Equally important in this framework is the context, communities, and environments within which families live where the impacts of ongoing injustices, discrimination, and inadequate resources based upon the social, racial, cultural,

[a] Georgetown University Center for Child and Human Development, 3300 Whitehaven Street NW #3300, Washington, DC 20007, USA; [b] Department of Pediatrics, University of California, Nurture Connection, 3333 California Street, San Francisco, CA 94118, USA; [c] Johnson Policy Consulting, Nurture Connection, VT
* Corresponding author. 3300 Whitehaven Street NW #3300, Washington, DC 20007.
E-mail address: dwwillis1950@gmail.com

Pediatr Clin N Am 71 (2024) 1027–1045
https://doi.org/10.1016/j.pcl.2024.07.011
pediatric.theclinics.com
0031-3955/24/

and historic status and public policies continue to disadvantage and burden some families and communities. These take a toll on parents, young children, and their relational health and well-being.[14–18]

Early relational health is foundational to building social emotional competences and future mental well-being. Decades of research across many related disciplines has irrefutably demonstrated that early relational experiences matter to optimal child development, neurodevelopment, and social emotional development for all children.[19–21] The impact of adverse childhood experiences on long-term health and mental health has likewise been well-established, especially in the absence of the buffering of safe, stable, and nurturing caregivers (**Box 1**).[1,22–26] And as research and understanding have progressed, the balancing protective effects of positive childhood experiences on health, mental health, and development, even in the face of adversity, have further emphasized the essential preventative influence of relational experiences.[27–29] With advances in the population-level survey data, the evidence is growing regarding the positive role of family resilience and social connections in support of early relational health, optimal development, mental health, and child flourishing.[30]

CHILD FLOURISHING AND FAMILY RESILIENCE AND CONNECTION

The concept of flourishing has been well-documented and defined in adults, but less has been known about flourishing and its correlates among children. Studies have shown that flourishing is distinct from the absence of physical or mental illness, and that flourishing can and does exist amid adversities, and health outcomes vary widely

Box 1
Putting principles into action: building an early relational health ecosystem

1. Nurturing caregiver-child interactions establish strong, meaningful, and enduring or consistent relationships and provide immediate and long-term benefits for both young children and their caregivers.
2. Simple and everyday human interactions are "good enough" early relational experiences.
3. Research and practice are strengthened by integrating family experience and cultural wisdom into the science of early childhood development.
4. Connectedness, belonging, and mattering are essential for parents.
5. The early relational health paradigm emphasizes the strengths and resources of parents and young children.
6. A social-ecological perspective enables a comprehensive focus on conditions, circumstances, and characteristics that advance or impede early relational health.
7. A broad range of helping professionals and community members can provide experiences, which promote early relational health.
8. Collaborative decision-making and power-sharing between families and early relational health professionals can lead to better outcomes for children and parents.
9. Early relational health embraces diversity of practices and knowledge and resists reductionism about human development.
10. A society built on respectful and equitable relationships is a society in which all young children and their families can thrive.

Data from Harper Browne, C., Li, J., O'Connor, C., Russo, J. E., & Willis, D.W. (2024). Putting Principles into Action: Building an Early Relational Health Ecosystem. Center for the Study of Social Policy and Nurture Connection. Pg. 5.

among individual exposed to similar levels of adversity.[31] Studies using attributes of child flourishing such as these show the reductions in risky health behaviors and future mental health issues, as well as the reduction of physical, mental, and social health problems as adults.[32] More recently, flourishing has become a topic explored in the annual National Survey of Children's Health (NSCH). For young children ages 0 to 5, the survey asks 4 questions that aim to capture curiosity and discovery about learning, resilience, attachment with parent, and contentment with life. The survey questions specifically ask: "How often: is this child affectionate and tender; does this child bounce back quickly when things do not go their way; does this child show interest and curiosity in learning new things; does this child smile and laugh? Responses of "Always" or "Usually" to the question indicate the child meets the flourishing item criteria. NSCH data show the nationwide prevalence of flourishing among children 0 to 5 was 78% (confidence interval [CI] 77.1–79.6) in 2022 (that is, meeting all 4 flourishing items).[33]

In addition, the NSCH and work of its Technical Expert Panel was used to establish the construct validity of a 3-item, parent reported Child Flourishing Index (CFI) along with a 6-item family resilience and connection index (FSCI), analyzing the relationship between the 2. The CFI items ask parents how well each of these 3 items describes their child: "shows interest and curiosity in learning new things"; "works to finish tasks he or she starts"; and "stays calm and in control when faced with a challenge." The 4-items of the family resilience index asked parents: "When your family faces problems, how often are you likely to": "talk together about what to do; work together to solve our problems; know we have strengths to draw on; and stay hopeful even in difficult times." Two additional items asked parents how well they "can share ideas or talk about things that really matter" with their child (parent-child connection) and how well they think they are "handling the day-to-day demands of raising children" (parent coping). These items together make up the FSCI.[30]

At each level of adverse childhood experience, household income and special health care needs, flourishing improves in a graded fashion with reported increases of family resilience and connection.[30] An especially strong association has been found between flourishing and the parent-child connection component of the family resilience and connection index score. This finding points to the importance of safe, stable, and nurturing relationships (SSNRs) and early relational health that supports optimal child development on the trajectory toward flourishing. By promoting positive childhood experiences and supporting the conditions for flourishing for all children, we have the opportunity to prevent poor mental health, even in face of adversity.[11,34]

OUR NATION'S CHILDREN ARE NOT FLOURISHING

The NSCH shows that nearly 1-quarter of our children are not flourishing.[33] In addition, the NSCH provides the only national- and state-level measure of young children's readiness to start kindergarten within the context of influential health, behavioral, family, and community-level factors.[35] Children who enter kindergarten healthy and ready to learn are more likely to meet academic milestones and future social, economic, and health outcomes over a lifespan. The NSCH assesses school readiness from parent and caregiver responses to 28 questions in 5 areas (domains): Early Learning Skills, Social-Emotional Development, Self-Regulation, Motor Development, and Health. Responses are scored according to age-appropriate developmental expectations as 'On Track', 'Emerging', or 'Needs Support'. In 2022, only 63.6% of 3 to 5 year old children were 'On Track' in 4 to 5 domains without needing support in any domain, with the remaining one-third of young children who are showing emerging skills or could benefit from additional supports.[35] More specifically, 72% were 'On Track' with self-regulation skills, and 82.9% 'On Track' with social-emotional development, as reported by parents. Yet, from the public health, life course, and population health perspectives, these losses of developmental potential are notable and are understood to be increasingly more difficult to rectify across the arc of development. The mechanisms, too, of these disparities are well-understood as arising from living in under-resourced and unsafe communities, racism and discrimination, family economic hardship, family stress and mental illness, trauma and adversity, and the absence of buffering relationships.[17,23,36–39] All of these challenges have the potential to disrupt the safe, stable, and nurturing experiences of the first 1000 days that contribute early relational health and future health, development, and well-being.

The children's mental health crisis, especially post-coronavirus disease 2019, has activated many sectors across mental health, public health, and medicine.[33,40–42] As articulated by Vivek Murthy, MD, United States (US) Surgeon General, loneliness, social isolation, and disconnection area major contributors to the current national mental health crisis.[43] One in 6 US children aged 2 to 8 y (17.4%) have a diagnosed mental, behavioral, or developmental disorder.[44] National surveys of families of young children are also articulating their family stress, loneliness, and hardships.[45,46] All of these data point to the importance of increasing the efforts of the public health and child health systems to support and ensure positive, strong, and nurturing relationships in the earliest years.

CHILD MENTAL WELL-BEING IS AN OUTCOME OF EARLY RELATIONAL HEALTH

Parent-child interactions are known to have impact on later mental and social well-being.[47–49] Studies of the quality of the parent-child interactions, the maternal sensitivity to their infants, and the impact of a secure attachment relationship have all contributed to our understanding of the importance of early nurturing relationships, early relational health, and later well-being outcomes.[19,50–53] In addition, challenges in early childhood social-emotional functioning seems be associated with later emerging mental health conditions.[32,54] One study showed that 40% of children entering school with relative vulnerabilities in social-emotional functioning are subsequently associated with early-onset mental health conditions.[55] Notably, many of these studies are limited by small sample sizes, participant homogeneity, and short time horizons that make scaling, population impacts, and public health guidance more challenging.

Recent analysis of the NCHS data has also demonstrated how social risks, relational risks, and their interactions early in life are associated with mental and behavioral health considerations among older children and youth.[34] Social risks are defined as serious economic hardship, food insufficiency, neighborhood violence, and racial discrimination. Relational risks are defined as the presence of multiple adverse childhood experiences, poor or fair parent/caregiver mental health, or high parental stress. In fact, there is a 4-fold difference in the prevalence of children's mental health conditions depending on the social and relational health risks they experience (**Fig. 1**). These new understandings compel the development and implementation of new approaches to both universal prevention and targeted interventions.

PEDIATRIC PRIMARY CARE PROVIDES NEAR UNIVERSAL ACCESS TO ALL CHILDREN

Pediatric primary health care is the only service sector that sees virtually all infants and young children before their primary school years through well-child visits, and thus offers the best opportunity for advancing promotion, prevention, and early intervention efforts to vast numbers of families to support their physical, developmental, and

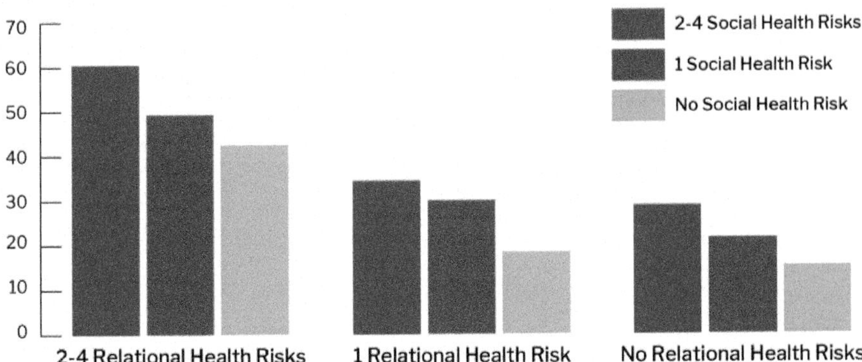

Fig. 1. Mental-emotional and behavioral conditions among children 3 to 17, by relational and social health risks. (*Data from* Bethell et al. Social and Relational Health Risks and Common Mental Health Problems Among US Children. Child Adolesc Psychiatric Clin N A,. 2022;31:45-70. https://doi.org/10.1016/j.chc.2021.08.001.)

social-emotional well-being. Although affected by recent disenrollments in Medicaid, 95% of the nation's young children had health coverage by January 2023. Notably, by that date, more than half of all children under age 18 were covered by Medicaid and the Children's Health Insurance Program (CHIP)[56] These all-time high coverage rates reflected federal and state policy protections for continuous coverage and, while final national data are not yet available, recent disenrollments are eroding coverage in many states.

The nation's approximately 34,870 primary care pediatricians[57] provide the majority of child health care for those families located within urban and suburban areas (where most US children reside), whereas about a 68% of the nation's approximately104,000 family physicians provide health care to children, more often located in disadvantaged communities or in rural and frontier areas.[58] Pediatricians provide the majority of the management of acute and chronic illnesses of children, while also trained to focus on prevention and promotion of health, development, and well-being of all children. Building on the latest research in neurodevelopment and early child development, the most recent edition of the American Academy of Pediatrics' (AAP's) *Bright Futures*—the nation's guide for quality child health care standards—strongly emphasizes the importance of early brain and child development, the social determinants of health (SDoH), and positive and supportive parent-child relationships to both the physical and mental health of children.[59] Hence, child health care is the key universal platform for supporting and promoting the foundations of health, development, and future well-being, capacities that are increasingly understood as outcomes of early relational experiences in the context of their environments.[60–62]

The AAP 2021 Policy Statement calls for a focus on the SSNRs in child health that buffers adversity and builds resilience that would galvanize a paradigm shift to reprioritize clinical activities, rewrite research agendas, and realign collective advocacy to promoting relational health in partnership with communities and families.[1] And the relational health framework challenges the entire pediatric community to adopt a public health approach that builds relational health by partnering with families and communities and redesigning systems that are integrated both vertically (by including primary, secondary, and tertiary preventions) and horizontally (by including public service sectors beyond health care). Vertically integrated approaches are founded on universal primary preventions (eg, promoting family resilience, social connections, and positive childhood experiences), with tiered, targeted interventions (eg, addressing parental depression, SDoHs), and indicated treatments (eg, dyadic therapy, parent-child interaction therapy) (**Fig. 2**). A public health approach to promote relational health should also be integrated horizontally (or across sectors) locally, and has been articulated as an aspirational as a Family-Centered Community Health System—an integrated, equitable community and child/family health system model to advance equity and ERH.[63] The key elements include:

1. A place-based approach for achieving population health with data that inform local decision-making.
2. A local, coordinated early childhood system that works to dismantle structural inequities.
3. High-performing medical homes that better support families.
4. Parent leadership networks that hold programs and services systems accountable.
5. Strategies that support ERH for improved life course outcomes.
6. Vibrant and robust family- and community-led networks that support positive experiences for children and families.

ADVANCING HIGH PERFORMING MEDICAL HOMES FOR YOUNG CHILDREN

For decades, the concept of a medical home has been advanced as an approach for delivery of comprehensive primary care that facilitates partnerships between patients, providers, and families.[64] A well-implemented and adequately financed medical home can help to achieve the triple aims of health care to improve the experience of care, improve population health, and reduce costs.[65–67] The AAP, as well as the US Department of Health and Human Services, Health Resources and Services Administration, Maternal and Child Health Bureau (HRSA-MCHB) and Centers for Medicare and Medicaid Services, all recommend that each child have a patient/family-centered medical home.

The AAP introduced the medical home concept for children in 1967.[68,69] As defined by the AAP and HRSA-MCHB, a pediatric medical home must be accessible, family-centered, continuous, comprehensive, coordinated, compassionate, and culturally effective.[70–73] For decades, these organizations, parent advocacy organizations, and other leaders in child health emphasized the importance of providing a medical home for children with special health care needs—defined as children who have or are at increased risk for chronic physical, developmental, behavioral, or emotional

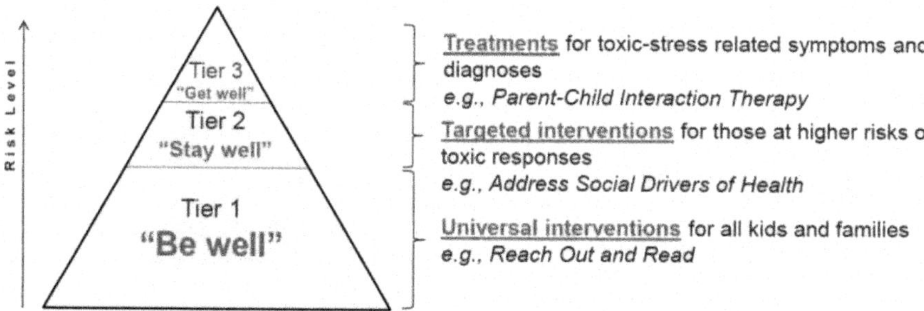

Fig. 2. Vertical integration: tiered supports for early relational health (ERH). (*Adapted from* Garner A, Yogman M, Health CoPAoCaF, Pediatrics SoDaB, Childhood CoE. Preventing Childhood Toxic Stress: Partnering With Families and Communities to Promote Relational Health. Pediatrics. 2021;148(2):e2021052582. https://doi.org/10.1542/peds.2021-052582.)

conditions and who require health and related services of a type or amount beyond that required by children generally.[74] This includes, but is not limited to, children with complex medical conditions.

The medical home has also been significantly associated with increased preventive care visits (adjusted odds ratio [aOR]: 1.32 [95% CI: 1.22–1.43]), decreased outpatient sick visits (aOR: 0.71 [95% CI: 0.66–0.76), and decreased emergency department sick visits (aOR: 0.70 [95% CI: 0.65–0.76]). It was associated with increased odds of "excellent/very good" child health according to parental assessment (aOR: 1.29 [95% CI: 1.15–1.45) and health-promoting behaviors such as being read to daily (aOR: 1.46 [95% CI: 1.13–1.89]), reported helmet use (aOR: 1.18 [95% CI: 1.03–1.34]), and decreased screen time (aOR: 1.12 [95% CI: 1.02–1.22]).[75] More recent recommendations and initiatives have focused on ensuring a medical home for all children.[75–78]

Over time, other governmental and medical professional organizations adopted the medical home concept for adult care as well. By 2007, the 4 major organizations representing primary care providers—AAP, American Academy of Family Physicians, American College of Physicians, and American Osteopathic Association—developed the "*Joint Principles of the Patient-Centered Medical Home (PCMH).*"[79] These organizations adopted the National Center for Quality Assurance (NCQA) criteria for PCMH as standards for practice for both children and adults and, under NCQA standards, practices can gain PCMH recognition (sometimes called certification).[80] An increasing body of literature identifies the key characteristics of a medical home or PCMH. Today, the shared principles are generally defined as delivering primary care that is: patient and family-centered, comprehensive, team-based, accessible, coordinated and committed to quality, safety, and equity.[81] Although not always included in lists of the attributes of the medical home, equity was identified as 1 of the 6 core dimensions of a high-performing, high-quality health care system in the landmark Institute of Medicine report *Crossing the Quality Chasm*.[82]

Despite the documented advantages of having a medical home and its promotion by governmental, professional, and family advocacy organizations, too few US children have a medical home. National performance on this measure is low and has not been substantially improving.[83] The NSCH composite measure for a medical home includes having: (1) a personal doctor or nurse, (2) a usual source for sick care, (3) family-centered care, (4) few problems getting connected to needed referral resources, and (5) effective care coordination when needed. The 2022 NSCH data show that less than half (47%) of US families with young children ages 0 to 5 reported that their children received care in a medical home. Rates of access vary by race/ethnicity. Among those under age 18, only 55% of White, non-Hispanic, 35% of Black non-Hispanic, 37% of Asian non-Hispanic, and 34% of Hispanic children having care that met the basic criteria for a medical home in 2022.[84]

A growing number of studies illuminate the disparities in access to a medical home.[85–88] Being uninsured, low income, in a home where English is not the primary household language, and/or a child of color all decrease the likelihood of having even a basic a medical home. Moreover, living in a community with higher levels of social vulnerability is also associated with less access to medical homes.[89–91] For example, living with the "pair of adverse childhood experiences (ACEs)"—that is, both ACEs based in the family and the community—creates greater challenges.[92–95] The medical home model has not consistently resulted in more equitable care for Black and Brown families, who are less likely to receive care that aligns with the principles of the medical home.[96–98] Studies also suggest that the current design and practice may not be effective in delivering health care to Hispanic children, particularly those in non-English speaking homes.[98,99] The prevalence of medical homes for American Indian/Alaska Native children (in 7 states reporting) was found to be low, despite being primarily funded by multiple federal programs.[100] Moreover, researchers have found that parental reports of their children having a medical home did not significantly reduce the negative association between unmet basic needs and excellent/very good child health, and one study concluded that "the AAP medical home concept, which was built upon fundamental tenets of primary care as currently constructed, may not be sufficient to attenuate the deleterious effects of unmet basic needs on low-income children's health."[101]

While all children should have access to a medical home, many families with young children in need additional support through what has been defined as a "high performing medical home."[102] A high performing medical home for young children would carry out functions beyond current standard practice and extend beyond the standard definition of the medical home. For children birth to 5 in particular, it would give more focus to promoting optimal development and to engaging parents of young children to achieve better outcomes.

Clearly improvement is needed to ensure equitable access to high quality, unbiased, and effective primary care for young children. As defined here and shown in **Fig. 3**, an advanced, team-based, high performing medical home for young children provides: (1) provides comprehensive, relational, and strengths-based well-child care based upon standards for well-child care included in AAP *Bright Futures* guidelines, (2) structures relational care coordination with care team members to connect with families and community resources, and (3) embeds or links to other services and supports. This is in line with the 2021 AAP statement calling for a paradigm shift to support relational health and AAP position on racism, which emphasize that children's primary care

Redesigned Well-Child Visits

- Holistic, **team-based care**
- Comprehensive **well- child visits** based on Bright Futures guidelines and EPSDT
- Family-centered, **strengths-based, relational**, holistic approaches
- **Recommended screening** for development, social-emotional health, maternal depression and social determinants of health (SDOH)
- Reach Out and Read as universal promotion

Relational Care Coordination

- **Routine** care coordination as part of medical home
- **Intensive care coordination** for more complex medical conditions or social risks
- **Relational care coordination staff** (e.g., community health workers, peer navigators)
- More **effective responses, completed referrals,** and **linkages** to community

Other Services and Enhanced Supports

- **Co-located programs in primary care** to promote ERH and development (e.g., DULCE, Healthy Steps, VIP)
- **Integrate mental health**
- **Families engaged** as advisors and partners
- **Referrals and/or linkages** to other services (e.g., home visiting, early intervention, dental care, early care and education, parent-child mental health therapy, nutrition programs)

Fig. 3. Design for the high performing medical home for young children. (*Adapted from* Willis DW, Paradis N, Johnson K. The paradigm shift to early relational health: A network movement. *Zero to Three*. 2022; 42(4):22-30; and Johnson K, Bruner C. *A Sourcebook on Medicaid's Role in Early Childhood: Advancing high performing medical homes and improving lifelong health*. Child and Family Policy Center. 2018. https://www.inchmarks.org/docs/pdfs_for_Medicaid_and EPSDT_page/SourcebookMEDICAIDYOUNGCHILDRENALL.pdf.)

providers need: sufficient time with patients and families, continuity of care and families, and the skills needed to form respectful, trusted, and collaborative relationships with families. Team-based care using strengths-based approaches have been shown to help in building trust and making care more acceptable and effective.

As a key component, a high performing medical home requires *enhanced, relational care coordination*, which most practices are not currently equipped to provide.[103] The need for enhanced, relational care coordination can be due to medical complexity or social complexity, and which disproportionately affect children covered by Medicaid or residing in medically-underserved and low-income communities. Such enhanced care coordination offers structured and effective efforts to engage with the family to identify needs and help secure services and supports to respond to families' needs. It involves a worker trained and skilled in family engagement, who must be recognized as an integral member of the medical home team. While the worker may be hired for their knowledge of and connections to the community being served, they must also have appropriate skills for fostering relationships. An increasing body of evidence supports the use of this type of care coordination to address concrete needs and social risks.[104–114]

Brunauer and Hayes describe advanced, team-based medical homes this way: "At the practice level, different initiatives have described these as "high performing medical homes,"[102] "whole child medical homes,"[115,116] and "relational health homes".[117] Such advanced medical homes share qualities of being team-based, family-driven, and community-connected. They offer care to families that is holistic, relational, strengths-based, preventive, and developmental. The focus of this approach to pediatric primary care is on optimizing all aspects of a young child's development—physical, cognitive, social-relational, and emotional-behavioral—in the context of the child's family, neighborhood, school, and community.

INTEGRATING EARLY RELATIONSHIP PRINCIPLES INTO PEDIATRIC PRIMARY CARE

In pediatric primary care, the early relationship between the caregiver and child forms the bedrock of optimal emotional, cognitive, and physical development. Pediatricians, as frontline health care providers, who see more than 90% of young children, are uniquely positioned to influence and support the development of these early relationships. By promoting secure attachments and promoting social emotional attunement early, pediatricians support nurturing connections and early relational health. This proactive approach aligns with the principles of preventive care, aiming to optimize developmental trajectories and overall health.

Tips for Pediatric Practices

- There are many ways to support ERH in practice that extend beyond incorporating developmental surveillance into routine visits to observing the caregiver-child interactions, providing concrete suggestions that build caregiver capacity and addressing social drivers of health.
- Pediatric practices should create physical environments that foster positive strength-based interactions. This includes designing family-friendly comfortable waiting areas that are welcoming and include spaces that encourage caregiver-child interaction. Educational materials on parenting can be made available. Clinics can consider having books that represent a diversity of cultures and languages, as well as colorful and inclusive signage.
- Pediatricians have the opportunity to express their interest in supporting parents in the growth of their relationships with their infants and young children. Starting

conversations about parent-child relationships at the earliest well-child visits may include such questions as:[118]

- What 3 words or phrases would you use to describe your relationship with your baby?
- What brings you the most joy in the relationship with your baby?
- What is your biggest fear about your relationship with your baby?

These are meant to be conversations and opportunities for parents to share their reflections on their developing relationships and offer the pediatrician a moment to signal of their ongoing interest.

- During routine visits, pediatricians should observe caregiver-child interactions to assess the quality of their relationship. This can be done through direct observation and the use of structured, objective, and validated screening tools such as the Ages and Stages Questionnaires (ASQs).[119] Observational assessments allow pediatricians to provide immediate, constructive feedback to caregivers, reinforcing positive behaviors and gently guiding improvements where necessary. Pediatricians can more frequently comment on what they are witnessing in the caregiver-child interaction making comments such as "every time you look at your baby, they smile at you," "I love the way that they want to give you hugs," and "I notice how they just keep looking at you."
- Providing caregivers with practical advice on fostering positive, strong, and nurturing relationships is crucial. This can include guidance on responsive feeding, soothing techniques, and promoting play. For example, a pediatrician notices that a father seems unsure how to engage with his 6-month-old during a visit. The pediatrician demonstrates simple games like peek-a-boo and explains how such simple interactions support social and emotional development. Another example is a mother who expresses concerns about her baby's frequent crying. The pediatrician discusses the concept of responsive feeding and soothing techniques, such as swaddling and gentle rocking, emphasizing the importance of responding to the baby's needs promptly to build trust and security. Providing a caregiver with practical advice on responsive parenting is essential to being attuned to their child's needs, recognizing and responding to cues, and engaging in play and other bonding activities.
- The well-baby visits are incredible opportunities for pediatricians can model positive interactions during examinations. This involves engaging the child with eye contact, smiles, and gentle touch, showing caregivers effective ways to connect with their child. During a check-up, a pediatrician smiles and talks softly to a toddler while conducting the examination. Engage in call and response and follow where the baby's interests in directing. The pediatrician then explains to the parents how these behaviors can engage, help soothe, and comfort their child, encouraging them to use similar techniques at home.
- Maternal mental health significantly affects early relationships. Using screening tools like the Edinburgh Postnatal Depression Scale (EPDS) during well-child visits is recommended in Bright Futures and helps to identify mothers at risk of depression, facilitating timely intervention.[120] When a depression screen result is positive, management will vary according to the degree of concern and need. For instance, if a caregiver completes the EPDS and scores high, indicating possible depression, the pediatrician can discuss these results, provides supportive resources such as a link to the local Baby Blues Networks, or the refer her back to her doctor and then ensure follow-up. The pediatrician also discusses how caregiver mood can affect their interactions with their baby and provides tips to strengthen their bond.

- Pediatric practices should establish strong connections with community-based resources such as food banks, housing programs early intervention programs, mental health services, and social support networks. These partnerships can provide comprehensive support to families, addressing a wide range of needs that impact early relational health. Screening for unmet basic needs and financial health has been consistently shown to reduce caregiver stress and improve child development.[121,122]
- Using designated care coordinators is part of a high-performing medical home and can facilitate community connections. For example, the FIND program is staffed by community health workers who have lived experience similar to the patient populations being served. They tailor their health education and resource and referral linkage to programs and activities that support children and families. The community health works are especially knowledgeable about referring to childcare organizations like Head Start, Regional Centers, parenting groups, diaper banks, and Women Infant and Child Programs. Research has demonstrated that care coordination leads to reduced emergency room visits, hospital stays, and improves child health.[104,105]
- Additionally, when high-performing medical homes address the financial health of families of young children, we see a reduction of caregiver stress and anxiety and improved child development. Programs such a Brilliant Baby provide financial coaching and seed funding for college saving accounts for children before the 5th birthday. Early child community health workers are trained to talk with families about the possibility of shifting a hope to an expectation of a college/vocational bound future. Treading out starting at 6 m from enrollment, children's ASQs improve, and caregivers feel more confident about the future.[123]

Beyond community health workers, building diverse and multidisciplinary teams across the community—including doulas, social workers, psychologists, early care and education teachers, and early intervention specialists—ensures comprehensive care for families facing complex social and medical challenges. This team approach can address a wide range of issues that impact early relationships. Many clinics have integrated behavioral health (BHI) models whereby mental health clinicians work alongside pediatricians and co-see families. In an ideal case, a pediatrician who is concerned about a child exhibiting behavioral concerns can refer to their mental health colleagues via BHI who can then provide short-term therapy, refer the family to an early intervention specialist and coordinates with a trauma-informed team to provide holistic support, including parenting workshops and mental health services.

BLOOM (Black Love Opportunity and Outcome Improvement in Medicine) is a Black Baby Equity Clinic at UCSF Benioff Children's Hospital in Oakland, CA.[124] BLOOM is changing the way early relational care is delivered to Black families in an environment that is safe, supportive, and respectful. This model is building from the awareness that Black physicians double the survival odds of Black infants and children.[125] At one location, families receive care from Black pediatricians, health educators, therapists, navigators, family support specialists and breastfeeding coaches, where relationally-centric care is a core value. Focusing to provide racially and culturally congruent care, their team seeks to address the needs and priorities of each patient and family, as well as the well-being of Black physicians and staff.

SUMMARY

Transforming pediatric practice to support early relational health requires a comprehensive, multifaceted approach. Integrating early relationship principles into pediatric primary care is a powerful strategy to enhance child development and health outcomes. By adopting a holistic, preventive approach that includes early identification, caregiver education, and support for families, pediatricians can play a pivotal role in fostering secure attachments and promoting lifelong well-being. Making the paradigm shift toward early relational health and transforming our practices into high-performing medical homes for young children is within reach—using emerging best practices, evidence-based models, and the Bright Futures guidelines in combination with respectful, strengths-based, and relational approaches. As frontline health care providers, pediatricians have the opportunity and responsibility to nurture the early relationships that form the foundation for a child's future success and family well-being.

CLINICS CARE POINTS

- Discussions with parents about ERH should begin as universal promotion activities in the earliest well-child visits
- Primary care staff can model relational health in their authentic and sensitive interactions with infants, toddlers, and youth
- Team-based care models offer many opportunities to advance relational health care
- Listen to and partner with families for their wisdom to guide the relational transformation of child health care.

DISCLOSURE

The authors have neither commercial nor financial conflicts of interest. Drs D.W. Willis, D. Long and K. Johnson are supported through Nurture Connection by the Einhorn Collaborative.

REFERENCES

1. Garner A, Yogman M, Committee on Psychosocial Aspects of Child and Family Health, et al. Preventing childhood toxic stress: partnering with families and communities to promote relational health. Pediatrics 2021;148(2). https://doi.org/10.1542/peds.2021-052582. e2021052582.
2. Willis D, Eddy JM. Early relational health: innovations in child health for promotion, screening and research. Infant Ment Health J 2022;43(3):361–72.
3. Roby E, Canfield C, Seery A, et al. Promotion of positive childhood experiences and early relational health in pediatric primary care: accumulating evidence. Academic Pediatrics 2024;25(2):201–3.
4. Dumitriu D, Lavallée A, Riggs JL, et al. Advancing early relational health: a collaborative exploration of a research agenda. Frontiers in Pediatrics 2023. https://doi.org/10.3389/fped.2023.1259022.
5. Johnson K, Nagle G and Willis D. State leadership and policy action to advance early relational health. Available at: https://nurtureconnection.org/resource/policy-early-relational-health/, (Accessed July 30 2024). 2023.
6. Li J and Ramirez T. Early relational health: a review of research, principles and perspectives. Available at: https://nurtureconnection.org/resource/early-relational-health-principles/, (Accessed July 30 2024). 2023.
7. Willis D, Paradis N, Johnson K. The paradigm shift to early relational health: a network movement. Washingon, DC: Zero to Three; 2022.

8. Center for the Study of Social Policy, Core story of early relational health: messaging guide. Available at: https://nurtureconnection.org/early-relational-health/core-story/, (Accessed July 30 2024). 2022.
9. Frameworks Institute. Building relationships: framing early relational health. Washington, DC: Frameworks Institute; 2020.
10. Donney JF, Ghandour RM, Kogan MD, et al. Family-centered care and flourishing in early childhood. Am J Prev Med 2022;63(5):743–50.
11. Crouch E, Radcliff E, Brown MJ, et al. Association between positive childhood experiences and childhood flourishing among US children. J Dev Behav Pediatr 2023;44(4):e255–62.
12. Luby JL. Early childhood nurturance and the sculpting of neurodevelopment. Am J Psychiatr 2020;177(9):795–6.
13. Osher D, Cantor P, Berg J, et al. Drivers of human development: how relationships and context shape learning and development. Appl Dev Sci 2022;24(1):6–36.
14. Jindal M, Trent M, Mistry KB. The intersection of race, racism, and child and adolescent health. Pediatr Rev 2022;43(8):415–25.
15. Johnson TJ. Intersection of bias, structural racism, and social determinants with health care inequities. Pediatrics 2020;146(2). https://doi.org/10.1542/peds.2020-003657. e2020003657.
16. National Academies of Sciences, Engineering, and Medicine. Closing the opportunity gap for young children. Washingon, DC: The National Academies Press; 2023. p. 386.
17. Jutte DP, Miller JL, Erickson DJ. Neighborhood adversity, child health, and the role for community development. Pediatrics 2015;135(Supplement_2):S48–57.
18. Sandel M, Faugno E, Mingo A, et al. Neighborhood-level interventions to improve childhood opportunity and lift children out of poverty. Academic Pediatrics 2016;16(3, Supplement):S128–35.
19. National Scientific Council on the Developing Child. 2004. Young children develop in an environment of relationships. Working Paper No. 1. Available at: http://www.developingchild.net. (Accessed August 17 2024).
20. National Academies of Sciences, Engineering, and Medicine, Division of Behavioral and Social Sciences and Education, Board on Children, Youth, and Families, Committee on Fostering Healthy Mental, Emotional, and Behavioral Development Among Children and Youth. Fostering Healthy Mental, Emotional, and Behavioral Development in Children and Youth: A National Agenda. Washington (DC): National Academies Press (US); 2019.
21. National Academies of Sciences, Engineering, and Medicine. Vibrant and healthy kids: aligning science, practice, and policy to advance health equity. Washingon, DC: The National Academies Press; 2019. p. 620.
22. Felitti VJ. Adverse childhood experiences and adult health. Academic Pediatrics 2009;9(3):131–2.
23. Shonkoff JP, Garner AS, Committee on Psychosocial Aspects of Child and Family Health, et al. The lifelong effects of early childhood adversity and toxic stress. Pediatrics 2012;129(1):e232–46.
24. Bethell CD, Simpson LA, Solloway MR. Child well-being and adverse childhood experiences in the United States. Academic Pediatrics 2017;17(7, Supplement):S1–3.
25. Burke NJ, Hellman JL, Scott BG, et al. The impact of adverse childhood experiences on an urban pediatric population. Child Abuse Negl 2011;35(6):408–13.
26. Larkin H, Shields J, Anda R. THe Health and Social Consequences of Adverse Childhood Experiences (ACE) across the lifespan: an introduction to prevention and intervention in the community. J Prev Interv Community 2012;40(4):263–70.

27. Bethell C, Jones J, Gombojav N, et al. Positive childhood experiences and adult mental and relational health in a statewide sample: associations across adverse childhood experiences levels. JAMA Pediatr 2019. https://doi.org/10.1001/jamapediatrics.2019.3007. e193007.
28. Sege R, Swedo EA, Burstein D, et al. Prevalance of positive childhood expereinces among adults - behavioral risk factor surveillance system, four states, 2015-2021. MMWR Morb Mortal Wkly Rep 2024;73:399–404.
29. Sege RD, Harper Browne C. Responding to ACEs with HOPE: health outcomes from positive experiences. Academic Pediatrics 2017;17(7, Supplement): S79–85.
30. Bethell CD, Gombojav N, Whitaker RC. Family resilience and connection promote flourishing among us children, even amid adversity. Health Aff 2019; 38(5):729–37.
31. VanderWeele TJ. On the promotion of human flourishing. Proc Natl Acad Sci USA 2017;114(31):8148–56.
32. Jones DE, Greenberg M, Crowley M. Early social-emotional functioning and public health: the relationship between kindergarten social competence and future wellness. Am J Publ Health 2015;105(11):2283–90.
33. Racine N, McArthur BA, Cooke JE, et al. Global prevalence of depressive and anxiety symptoms in children and adolescents during COVID-19: A Meta-analysis. JAMA Pediatr 2021. https://doi.org/10.1001/jamapediatrics.2021.2482.
34. Bethell C, Garner A, Gombojav N, et al. Social and relational health risks and common mental health problems among US children. Child Adolesc Psychiatr Clin N Am 2022;31(1):45–70.
35. National Survey of Children's Health: School Readiness, 2022. Data Brief. Available at: https://mchb.hrsa.gov/sites/default/files/mchb/data-research/2023-nsch-hrtl-brief-oct-2023.pdf, (Accessed July 30 2024). 2023.
36. Garner AS, Shonkoff JP, Committee on Psychosocial Aspects of Child and Family Health, et al. Early childhood adversity, toxic stress, and the role of the pediatrician: translating developmental science into lifelong health. Pediatrics 2012; 129(1):e224–31.
37. Wilkerson A, Laurore J, Maxfield E, et al. Racism creates inequities in maternal and child health, even before birth. Washingon, DC: Childs Trends; 2021.
38. Shonkoff JP, Slopen N, Williams DR. Early childhood adversity, toxic stress, and the impacts of racism on the foundations of health. Annu Rev Publ Health 2021. https://doi.org/10.1146/annurev-publhealth-090419-101940.
39. Clark K, Cahill R, Ansell D. Early Childhood Development and the Role of Neighbourhood Hubs for Supporting Children's Development and Wellbeing in Disadvantaged Communities: A Review of the Literature (2022). Life Course Centre Working Paper No. 2022-11, Available at: http://dx.doi.org/10.2139/ssrn.4118008. (Accessed July 30 2024).
40. The US Surgeon General's Advisory. Protecting Youth Mental Health. 2021. Washington, DC. Available at: https://www.hhs.gov/sites/default/files/surgeon-general-youth-mental-health-advisory.pdf. (Accessed July 30 2024).
41. Ghandour RM, Sherman LJ, Vladutiu CJ, et al. Prevalence and treatment of depression, anxiety, and conduct problems in US children. J Pediatr 2019; 206:256–67.e3.
42. US Department of Health and Human Services, US Department of Education and US Department of Justice, Report of the Surgeon general's conference on children's mental heatlh: a national action agenda, 2000, US Department of Health

and Human Services; Washington, DC. Available at: https://www.ncbi.nlm.nih.gov/books/NBK44233/. (Accessed July 30 2024).
43. The U.S. surgeon general's advisory on the healing effects of social connection and community. Our epidemic of loneliness and isolation. Available at: https://www.hhs.gov/sites/default/files/surgeon-general-social-connection-advisory.pdf. (Accessed July 30 2024). 2023.
44. Center for Disease Control (CDC), Children's Mental Health: data and statistics. Available at: https://www.cdc.gov/childrensmentalhealth/data.html. (Accessed July 30 2024).
45. Capita. The ties that bind and nurture: results of the NC social solidarity survey. Available at: https://www.capita.org/capita-ideas/2022/7/25/new-report-the-ties-that-bind-and-nurture. (Accessed July 30 2024). 2022.
46. Fisher P, Lombardi J and Kendall-Taylor N. A year in the life of a pandemic: what we've learned listening to family voices. Medium. Available at: https://medium.com/rapid-ec-project/a-year-in-the-life-of-a-pandemic-4c8324dda56b. (Accessed July 30 2024).
47. Bernier A, Calkins SD, Bell MA. Longitudinal associations between the quality of mother–infant interactions and brain development across infancy. Child Dev 2016;87(4):1159–74.
48. Marquis-Brideau C, Bernier A, Cimon-Paquet C, et al. Trajectory of quality of mother-child interactions: prospective links with child socioemotional functioning. Soc Dev 2022. https://doi.org/10.1111/sode.12644.
49. Feldman R, Bamberger E, Kanat-Maymon Y. Parent-specific reciprocity from infancy to adolescence shapes children's social competence and dialogical skills. Attach Hum Dev 2013;15(4).
50. Arguz Cildir D, Ozbek A, Topuzoglu A, et al. Association of prenatal attachment and early childhood emotional, behavioral, and developmental characteristics: a longitudinal study. Infant Ment Health J 2019. https://doi.org/10.1002/imhj.21822.
51. Groh AM, Fearon RMP, Ijzendoorn MH, et al. Attachment in the early life course: meta-analytic evidence for its role in socioemotional development. Child Development Perspectives 2017;11(1):70–6.
52. Murphy YE, Zhang X, Gatzke-Kopp L. The developmental cascade of early parenting, emergence of executive functioning, and emotional symptoms across childhood. Infant Ment Health J 2021. https://doi.org/10.1002/imhj.21913.
53. Behrendt HF, Scharke W, Herpertz-Dahlmann B, et al. Like mother, like child? Maternal determinants of children's early social-emotional development. Infact Ment Health J 2019. https://doi.org/10.1002/imhj.21765.
54. Thomson KC, Richardson CG, Samji H, et al. Early childhood social-emotional profiles associated with middle childhood internalizing and wellbeing. J Appl Dev Psychol 2021;76:101301.
55. Thomson KC, Richardson CG, Gadermann AM, et al. Association of childhood social-emotional functioning profiles at school entry with early-onset mental health conditions. JAMA Netw Open 2019;2(1):e186694.
56. Georgetown University Center for Children and Families. Available at: https://ccf.georgetown.edu/2017/03/03/medicaid-fact-sheets/. (Accessed December 5 2020).
57. US Bureau of Labor Statistics. Available at: https://www.bls.gov/oes/current/oes291221.htm. (Accessed May 30 2024).

58. Makaroff LA, Xierali IM, Petterson SM, et al. Factors influencing family physicians' contribution to the child health care workforce. Ann Fam Med 2014; 12(5):427–31.
59. Hagan J, Shaw JS, Duncan PM, editors. Bright futures: guidelines for health supervision of infants, children and adolescents. 4th edition. Itasca, IL: American Academy of Pediatrics; 2017.
60. Frosch C, Schoppe-Sullivan S, O'Banion D. Parenting and child development: a relational health perspective. Am J Lifestyle Med 2019;19(4).
61. Doyle S, Chavez S, Cohen S and Morrison S. Fostering Social and Emotional Health through Pediatric Primary Care: Common Treads to Transform Practice and Systems. Center for the Study of Social Policy, 2019. Available at: https://cssp.org/resource/fostering-social-emotional-health/. (Accessed July 30 2024).
62. Shah PE, Muzik M, Rosenblum KL. Optimizing the early parent–child relationship: windows of opportunity for parents and pediatricians. Curr Probl Pediatr Adolesc Health Care 2011;41(7):183–7.
63. Willis D. Advancing a family-centered community health system: a community agenda focused on child health care, early relationships, and equity. Washington, DC: Center for the Study of Social Policy; 2020.
64. Agency for Healthcare Research and Quality, U.S. Department of Health and Human Services. Defining the Patient Centered Medical Home (PCMH). Available at: https://pcmh.ahrq.gov/page/defining-pcmh. (Accessed July 30 2024).
65. Berwick D, Nolan T, Whittington J. The triple aim: care, health and cost. Health Aff 2008;27(3):759–69.
66. Price J, Brandt ML, Hudak ML, et al. Principles of financing the medical home for children. Pediatrics 2020;145(1). https://doi.org/10.1542/peds.2019-3451.
67. Bodenheimer T, Sinsky C. From triple to quadruple aim: care of the patient requires care of the provider. Ann Fam Med 2014;12(6):573.
68. Sia C, Tonniges TF, Osterhus E, et al. History of the medical home concept. Pediatrics 2004;113(5 Supplement):1473–8.
69. Dickens M, Green J, Kohrt A, et al. The medical home. Pediatrics 1992; 90(5):774.
70. American Academy of Pediatrics National Resource Center for Patient/Family-Centered Medical Home. Available at: https://medicalhomeinfo.aap.org/Pages/default.aspx. (Accessed July 30 2024).
71. MCH Library at Georgetown University. MCH Evidence for MCH Programs. Available at: https://www.mchevidence.org/tools/npm/11-medical-home.php. (Accessed July 30 2024).
72. American Academy of Pediatric, Medical Home. Available at: https://www.aap.org/en-us/professional-resources/practice-transformation/medicalhome/Pages/home.aspx. (Accessed July 30 2024).
73. McPherson M, Arango P, Fox H, et al. A new definition of children with special health care needs. Pediatrics 1998;102(1 Pt 1):137–40.
74. Maternal and Child Health Bureau, Children and Youth with Special Health Care Needs.(CYSHCN). Available at: https://mchb.hrsa.gov/programs-impact/focus-areas/children-youth-special-health-care-needs-cyshcn#i. (Accessed July 30 2024).
75. Long WE, Bauchner H, Sege RD, et al. The value of the medical home for children without special health care needs. Pediatrics 2012;129(1):87–98.
76. Lichstein JC, Ghandour RM, Mann MY. Access to the medical home among children with and without special health care needs. Pediatrics 2018;142(6). https://doi.org/10.1542/peds.2018-1795.

77. Akobirshoev I, Parish S, Mitra M, et al. Impact of medical home on health care of children with and without special health care needs: update from the 2016 National Survey of Children's Health. Matern Child Health J 2019;23(11):1500–7.
78. Hadland SE, Long WE. A systematic review of the medical home for children without special health care needs. Matern Child Health J 2014;18(4):891–8.
79. American Academy of Family Physicians, American Academy of Pediatrics, American College of Physicians, American Osteopathic Association. Available at: https://www.aafp.org/dam/AAFP/documents/practice_management/pcmh/initiatives/PCMHJoint.pdf. (Accessed July 30 2024).
80. National Committee on Quality Assurance (NCQA) Patient Centered Medical Home. Available at: https://www.ncqa.org/programs/health-care-providers-practices/patient-centered-medical-home-pcmh/. (Accessed July 30 2024).
81. Primary Care Collaborative. Defining the medical home. Available at: https://www.pcpcc.org/about/medical-home. (Accessed July 30 2024).
82. Institute of Medicine (US) Committee on Quality of Health Care in America. Crossing the Quality Chasm: A New Health System for the 21st Century. Washington DC; National Academies Press, 2001. Available at: https://www.ncbi.nlm.nih.gov/books/NBK222274/. (Accessed July 30 2024).
83. Bethell CD, Read D, Brockwood K, et al. Using existing population-based data sets to measure the American Academy of Pediatrics definition of medical home for all children and children with special health care needs. Pediatrics 2004; 113(5 Suppl):1529–37.
84. Child and Adolescent Health Measurement Initiative (CAHMI). National Survey of Children's Health (NSCH). Available at: www.childhealthdata.org. (Accessed July 30 2024).
85. Diao K, Tripodis Y, Long WE, et al. Socioeconomic and racial disparities in parental perception and experience of having a medical home, 2007 to 2011-2012. Acad Pediatr 2017;17(1):95–103.
86. Zickafoose JS, Davis MM. Medical home disparities are not created equal: differences in the medical home for children from different vulnerable groups. J Health Care Poor Underserved 2013;24(3):1331–43.
87. Guerrero AD, Rodriguez MA, Flores G. Disparities in provider elicitation of parents' developmental concerns for US children. Pediatrics 2011;128(5):901–9.
88. Berdahl TA, Friedman BS, McCormick MC, et al. Annual report on health care for children and youth in the United States: trends in racial/ethnic, income, and insurance disparities over time, 2002-2009. Acad Pediatr 2013;13(3):191–203.
89. Bell N, Wilkerson R, Mayfield-Smith K, et al. Community social determinants and health outcomes drive availability of patient-centered medical homes. Health Place 2021;67:102439.
90. Jones RM, Anyigbo C, Morris H, et al. Does a medical home buffer the association between child poverty and poor health? J Health Care Poor Underserved 2021;32(4):1935–48.
91. Stevens GD, Seid M, Pickering TA, et al. National disparities in the quality of a medical home for children. Matern Child Health J 2010;14(4):580–9.
92. Ellis W, Dietz W. A new framework for addressing adverse childhood and community experiences: the building community resilience model. Academic Pediatrics 2017;17(7):S86–93.
93. Ellis W. A pair of ACEs tree, Available at: https://publichealth.gwu.edu/sites/g/files/zaxdzs4586/files/2023-06/resource-description_pair-of-aces-tree.pdf. (Accessed July 30 2024).

94. Koita K, Long D, Hessler D, et al. Development and implementation of a pediatric adverse childhood experiences (ACEs) and other determinants of health questionnaire in the pediatric medical home: a pilot study. PLoS One 2018; 13(12):e0208088.
95. Cohen ARKK, Johnson M, Michelson KN, et al. Shared decision-making for families facing adversity and the role of the medical home. Pediatrics 2022;149(1 Meeting Abstracts Feb 2022):69.
96. Liljenquist K, Coker T. Transforming well-child care to meet the needs of families at the intersection of racism and poverty. Academic Pediatrics 2021;21(8, Supplement):S102–7.
97. Weller BE, Faubert SJ, Ault AK. Youth access to medical homes and medical home components by race and ethnicity. Matern Child Health J 2020;24(2): 241–9.
98. Guerrero AD, Zhou X, Chung PJ. How well is the medical home working for latino and black children? Matern Child Health J 2018;22(2):175–83.
99. Cordova-Ramos EG, Tripodis Y, Garg A, et al. Linguistic disparities in child health and presence of a medical home Among United States Latino Children. Acad Pediatr 2022;22(5):736–46.
100. Barradas DT, Kroelinger CD, Kogan MD. Medical home access among American Indian and Alaska Native children in 7 states: National Survey of Children's Health. Matern Child Health J 2012;16(Suppl 1):S6–13.
101. Webb R, Whitham A, Tripodis Y, et al. Does parental report of having a medical home attenuate the negative association between unmet basic needs and health for low-income children? Glob Pediatr Health 2020;7. https://doi.org/10.1177/2333794x20985805. 2333794x20985805.
102. Johnson K, & Bruner C. A Sourcebook on Medicaid's Role in Early Childhood: Advancing High Performing Medical Homes and Improving Lifelong Health. Child and Family Policy Center; Des Moines, IA, 2018. Available at: www.cfpciowa.org. (Accessed July 30 2024).
103. Bruner C. Building a relational health workforce for young children: a framework for improving child well-being. Child & Family Policy Center, Des Moines, IA: InCK Marks Working Paper Series; 2021.
104. Gottlieb LM, Hessler D, Long D, et al. Effects of social needs screening and in-person service navigation on child health: a randomized clinical trial. JAMA Pediatr 2016;170(11):e162521.
105. Pantell MS, Hessler D, Long D, et al. Effects of in-person navigation to address family social needs on child health care utilization: a randomized clinical trial. JAMA Netw Open 2020;3(6):e206445.
106. Chung EK, Siegel BS, Garg A, et al. Screening for social determinants of health among children and families living in poverty: a guide for clinicians. Curr Probl Pediatr Adolesc Health Care 2016;46(5):135–53.
107. Arbour M, Fico P, Atwood S, et al. Benefits of a universal intervention in pediatric medical homes to identify and address health-related social needs: an observational cohort study. Academic Pediatrics 2022;22(8):1328–37.
108. Germán M, Alonzo JK, Williams IM, et al. Early childhood referrals by healthysteps and community health workers. Clin Pediatr (Phila) 2023;62(4):321–8.
109. Coker TR, Liljenquist K, Lowry SJ, et al. Community health workers in early childhood well-child care for medicaid-insured children: a randomized clinical trial. JAMA 2023. https://doi.org/10.1001/jama.2023.7197.

110. Hurst R, Liljenquist K, Lowry SJ, et al. A parent coach–led model of well-child care for young children in low-income communities: protocol for a cluster randomized controlled trial. JMIR Res Protoc 2021;10(11):e27054.
111. Mimila NA, Chung PJ, Elliott MN, et al. Well-child care redesign: a mixed methods analysis of parent experiences in the PARENT Trial. Academic Pediatrics 2017;17(7):747–54.
112. Coker TR, Chacon S, Elliott MN, et al. A parent coach model for well-child care among low-income children: a randomized controlled trial. Pediatrics 2016; 137(3):e20153013.
113. Garg A, Brochier A, Tripodis Y, et al. A social care system implemented in pediatric primary care: a cluster RCT. Pediatrics 2023;152(2). e2023061513.
114. Messmer E, Brochier A, Joseph M, et al. Impact of an on-site versus remote patient navigator on pediatricians' referrals and families' receipt of resources for unmet social needs. J Prim Care Community Health 2020;11. https://doi.org/10.1177/2150132720924252. 215013272092425.
115. Gratale DJ, Counts NZ, Hogan L, et al. Accountable communities for health for children and families: approaches for catalyzing and accelerating success. NAM Perspectives Discussion paper; 2020.
116. Whole Child Health Alliance. Key Elements of Whole Child Health Models. Available at: https://www.nemours.org/content/dam/nemours/nemoursorg/en/documents/whole-child-health-alliance-key-elements.pdf. (Accessed July 30 2024).
117. Bruner CH and Hayes M. Federal Health Policy Requires Child Health Investment Focus, Health Affairs Forefront, 2023. Available at: https://www.healthaffairs.org/content/forefront/federal-health-policy-requires-child-health-investment-focus 2023. (Accessed July 30, 2024).
118. Department of Health and Social Care. UK. Reflecting on parent-infant relationships: A practitioner's guide to starting conversations. Available at: https://www.gov.uk/government/publications/parent-infant-relationships-starting-conversa tions-practitioner-guide/reflecting-on-parent-infant-relationships-a-practitioners-guide-to-starting-conversations, (Accessed July 30 2024). 2024.
119. Squires J, Bricker D, Heo K, et al. Ages & Stages Questionnaires, 3rd edition (ASQ-3): a parent-completed child monitoring system. Bookes Publishing. Available at: www.products.brookespublishing.com. (Accessed July 30 2024).
120. Cox JL, Holden JM, Sagovsky R. Detection of postnatal depression. Development of the 10-item Edinburgh Postnatal Depression Scale. Br J Psychiatry 1987;150:782–6.
121. Dworkin PH, Garg A. Considering approaches to screening for social determinants of health. Pediatrics 2019;144(4):e20192395.
122. Chung EK, Siegel BS, Garg A, et al. Screening for social determinants of health among children and families living in poverty: a guide for clinicians. Curr Probl Pediatr Adolesc Health Care 2016;46(5):135–53.
123. Oakland Promise. Available at: https://oaklandpromise.org/. (Accessed July 30 2024).
124. Benioff Children's Hospital, BLOOM: Black Love Opportunity and Outcome Improvement in Medicine. Available at: https://bloomclinic.ucsf.edu/. (Accessed July 30 2024).
125. Greenwood BN, Hardeman RR, Huang L, et al. Physician–patient racial concordance and disparities in birthing mortality for newborns. Proc Natl Acad Sci USA 2020;117(35):21194.

Motivational Interviewing in Pediatric Mental Health

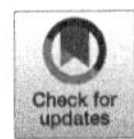

Rachel B. Herbst, PhD[a,b,c,*], Alexandra M.S. Corley, MD, MPH[b,c,1], Emily McTate, PhD[d,e,2], Julie M. Gettings, PhD[f,g,3]

KEYWORDS

• Motivational interviewing • Behavior change • Mental health • Primary care • Culturally-responsive care • Shared decision-making • Communication

KEY POINTS

- Motivational interviewing is an effective way of communicating with children and families to support behavior change related to a wide variety of presenting concerns.
- Motivational interviewing aligns with the core values of pediatric primary care, including partnership with families, health promotion, and cultural responsiveness.
- Pediatric clinicians can use motivational interviewing to enhance their assessment, management, and triaging of behavioral and mental health concerns.

INTRODUCTION

Motivational interviewing (MI), a conversational style intended to promote growth and change,[1] has been incorporated into various aspects of pediatrics over the past decade. MI may be considered an intervention that is primarily used by mental health

[a] Division of Behavioral Medicine and Clinical Psychology, Cincinnati Children's Hospital Medical Center, MLC 3015, 3333 Burnet Avenue, Cincinnati, OH 45229, USA; [b] Department of Pediatrics, College of Medicine, University of Cincinnati College of Medicine, 3230 Eden Avenue, Cincinnati, OH 45267, USA; [c] Division of General and Community Pediatrics, Cincinnati Children's Hospital Medical Center, 3333 Burnet Avenue, Cincinnati, OH 45229, USA; [d] Division of Child and Adolescent Psychiatry and Psychology, Department of Psychiatry and Psychology, Mayo Clinic, 200 1st Street Southwest, Rochester, MN 55906, USA; [e] Department of Pediatric and Adolescent Medicine, Mayo Clinic, Mayo Clinic College of Medicine and Science, 200 1st Street Southwest, Rochester, MN 55905, USA; [f] Department of Child and Adolescent Psychiatry and Behavioral Sciences, Children's Hospital of Philadelphia, 4601 Market Street, Third Floor, Philadelphia, PA 19139, USA; [g] Department of Clinical Psychiatry, Perelman School of Medicine, University of Pennsylvania, 3400 Civic Center Boulevard, Philadelphia, PA 19104, USA

[1] Present address: 3333 Burnet Avenue, MLC 7035, Cincinnati, OH 45229.

[2] Present address: 200 First Street SW, Rochester, MN 55905.

[3] Present address: 3500 Civic Center Boulevard, HUB-12594, Philadelphia, PA 19104.

* Corresponding author. MLC 3015, 3333 Burnet Avenue, Cincinnati, OH 45229.

E-mail address: rachel.herbst@cchmc.org

Twitter: @DrAlexCorley (A.M.S.C.); @jmgettings (J.M.G.)

Pediatr Clin N Am 71 (2024) 1047–1058

https://doi.org/10.1016/j.pcl.2024.07.012 pediatric.theclinics.com

0031-3955/24/

providers; however, it can be effectively used by a wide array of people working in helping professions, including pediatric clinicians. MI is among the most effective approaches to supporting behavior change in patients for a variety of presenting concerns.[2] Meta-analyses support the impact of MI in addressing a wide array of problem areas, including increasing health behaviors, promoting treatment adherence, increasing positive parenting practices, treating substance use disorder, decreasing risky behavior, and supporting emotional well-being.[2–4]

The collaborative, goal-oriented communication style of MI enables diverse applications and alignment with core values of pediatrics. Regardless of the presenting concern, MI focuses on identifying and strengthening an individual's personal "motivation for and commitment to a specific goal by eliciting and exploring the person's own reasons for change within an atmosphere of acceptance and compassion."[5] This article will outline the core components of MI, the inherent cultural responsiveness of MI, and therefore the broad applicability of MI to concerns in primary care, especially regarding mental and behavioral health.

DISCUSSION: WHAT IS MOTIVATIONAL INTERVIEWING?

Spirit of Motivational Interviewing

The foundation of MI is the "spirit" of the approach, which includes a genuine and helping-focused way of being with patients. Aligned with client-centered therapy[6] and positive psychology,[7] the spirit of MI reflects the idea that people are knowledgeable experts about themselves, and with skillful encouragement from pediatric clinicians, they are likely to grow in a positive way. Pediatric clinicians are called to be open, calm, and compassionate while resisting the natural urge to fix or correct a perceived problem.[1] In addition to the technical skills, the spirit of MI is revered as part of the process of promoting behavior change.

The MI spirit includes 4 elements: partnership, acceptance, compassion, and empowerment. For example, it is crucial that pediatric clinicians acknowledge their own biases and attitudes that may conflict with collaboration. More specifically, pediatric clinicians are encouraged to be mindful of implicit and explicit communication that minimizes power and privilege differences to promote an effective *partnership*. Pediatric clinicians are encouraged to *accept* the patient's attitudes, behaviors, and readiness to change—even if they conflict with the pediatric clinician's or medical team's own intentions. Similarly, *compassion* includes giving full priority to the well-being and interests of a patient rather than the interest of the pediatric clinician or others. Pediatric clinicians are called to promote *empowerment* by evoking motivation for goals and encouraging patient autonomy with decision-making.

Tasks of Motivational Interviewing

When using MI, Miller and Rollnick[1] delineate specific tasks that typically occur in conversations about change. The 4 tasks of MI are engaging, focusing, evoking, and planning. Although they may occur in a linear manner, it is also possible that the tasks overlap and blend with each other. *Engaging* involves empathic listening and establishing mutual respect and trust. Once this partnership is established, *focusing* means being deliberately directional about the purpose of the helping relationship. This may include establishing goals for the conversation as well as long-term goals for your work together. *Evoking* involves eliciting reasons for a patient making a change. Pediatric clinicians are challenged to notice and highlight *change talk* or any patient language that indicates movement toward their chosen target change behavior. This differs from *sustain talk*, which is a language that supports the status quo behavior.

In the evoking task, pediatric clinicians can skillfully invite the patient to consider and strengthen their own reasons why to make a change. *Planning* includes outlining the steps of how to make a change and is considered an ongoing discussion and process.

Core Skills

Effective practice of MI includes uses of 4 core communication skills, often abbreviated by the acronym OARS, including open questions, affirming, reflecting, and summarizing. *Open questions* invite more conversation, such as, "What have you tried so far in order to take your medicine more regularly?" *Affirming* involves hearing and then genuinely naming what you view as a positive-specific behavior (simple affirmation) or enduring strength (complex affirmation) of the person. This could include commenting on what they told you in your session ("You were really thoughtful in how you approached that problem.") or a characteristic they have shown ("You're a fighter who always finds a way to make things work."). *Reflections* demonstrate understanding of a person's statement and can be used to build rapport by showing that you are listening and attempting to understand them ("You're feeling overwhelmed about how to get to all of the appointments."). *Summaries* are a collection of reflections that are used to recount what was heard. They can be used to consolidate information and check if something is missing or ought to be discussed further. Commonly, after summarizing, the pediatric clinician may ask, "What else?" to allow for the person to have space to discuss anything additional.

Two additional skills that can be useful in an MI approach are ask-offer-ask as well as use of rulers for gauging patient preferences. *Ask-offer-ask* involves (1) asking the patient what they know already about a topic, (2) affirming accurate or helpful information while offering additional information with permission, and (3) asking patients to reflect on the new information offered. When evoking information from patients, it is sometimes helpful to use *rulers* to measure, importance, ability, or confidence. In doing so, the pediatric clinician may ask, "On a scale from 0 to 10, in which 0 is not important at all and 10 is extremely important, how important is it for you to make this change?" Once a number is stated, the pediatric clinician can then prompt why a lower number was not chosen in order to potentially generate further reflection or change talk (eg, "What made you chose a 5 and not a 2?").

As pediatric clinicians apply MI, there may be a tendency to focus solely on using MI skills to improve adherence, such as primarily focusing on open questions or reflections. We caution pediatric clinicians that overfocusing on skills often occurs at the sacrifice of the spirit of MI. In fact, learners of MI may be vulnerable to delays in conversation with a patient or diminished rapport while attempting to be overly skillful in their communication. We encourage pediatric clinicians to focus on the spirit of MI and how they are interacting with patients rather than the exact words they are saying. The OARS skills used in MI are intended as a vehicle to translate the spirit of MI into practice—not as a stringent approach to communication.

APPLICATION: WHY USE MOTIVATIONAL INTERVIEWING FOR MENTAL AND BEHAVIORAL HEALTH CONCERNS IN PRIMARY CARE?

Pediatric clinicians often have the unique privilege of longitudinal relationships with patients and their caregivers. This provides a port of entry to join with the family around their values and goals for their child. Ensuring alignment with the family's goals requires the pediatric clinician to engage in culturally-responsive care and to feel comfortable and confident in guiding the family through concerns about a wide variety of presenting concerns, including mental and behavioral health symptoms.

Culturally-Responsive Care

MI is inherently culturally responsive. Recognition and respect of a patient's lived experiences are core features of MI and culturally-responsive care. This lens enables pediatric clinicians to recognize how structural and systemic inequities, perpetuated throughout health care, differentially impact patients. For example, the hierarchy inherent in the pediatric clinician–patient relationship can pose barriers to collaborative decision-making, especially for people who have had historical experiences in which complying with hierarchies has been protective. This can cause a domino effect whereby patients are hesitant to assert their own agenda or discuss barriers to implementing the pediatric clinician's plan. For example, when a patient follows up and has not made recommended changes, patients are frequently labeled as "noncompliant" and both patients and pediatric clinicians may feel frustrated, placing the family at risk of decreasing their trust in the health care environment. MI can help to mitigate the impact of these inequities at the patient–pediatric clinician level. **Table 1** summarizes these considerations for culturally responsive care and MI-driven strategies for mitigation.

Miller and Rollnick,[1] codevelopers of MI, described how commitment to the use of MI transitions a pediatric clinician's conceptualization of MI from a strategy employed for specific presenting concerns to a "way of being." This means that the pediatric clinician integrates the values of MI, including a nonjudgmental approach that values empowerment and autonomy, into their professional (and often personal) identity.

Table 1
Cultural responsiveness in motivational interviewing

Considerations for Culturally Responsive Care	How MI Can Mitigate Impact
Patient–pediatric clinician hierarchy	• Explicit discussion about pediatric clinician's role as a guide • Affirming the value of the patient/family's lived experience and their expertise in their own lives • Collaborative agenda setting
Individualized focus, limited awareness of psychosocial stressors	• Understanding patient/family values and motivation • Appreciation of how presenting concerns, strengths, and barriers to behavior change relate to psychosocial and cultural factors (eg, mood is impacted by events experienced by the entire family system)
Implicit bias	• Intentional recognition of both pediatric clinician and patient/family values and motivations • Opportunity to view behavior through lens of strengths, capabilities, and patient/family autonomy
Unrecognized values within health care setting	• Explicit acknowledgment of system/pediatric clinician values (eg, being on time, communicating effectively, deference to the medical expertise of the pediatric clinician, adherence to recommendations), and how these impact patient care

Importance in Primary Care

Primary care seeks to meet a variety of health needs and goals, tackle both preventive care and disease management/treatment, develop long-term relationships with patients and families, and accomplish these goals with a posture of cultural humility.[8] MI skills are an important part of the toolkit for a pediatric clinician and can provide an essential framework for discussing behavior change with patients. The values of MI are aligned with the values of a pediatric clinician, including compassion, trust, and patient-centeredness. MI empowers individual patients and their families to be the drivers of change that can improve quality of life. MI skills may help a pediatric clinician identify a patient's priorities, build their self-efficacy, mitigate barriers and sustain healthy behaviors.

MI techniques are applicable to everyday clinical encounters, not just a theory or concept. As such, these are skills that must be learned and sustained through regular skill development and practice. Awareness of one's own biases, including preconceived expectations on capacity and timing for change, is critical. Frequent reflective practice can be useful alongside MI to ensure that one's deployment of MI skills focuses primarily on the goals and desires of patients and families, and less on the motivations of individual pediatric clinicians.

While the evidence base of MI is clear, it is not an approach that is guaranteed to work in all pediatric primary care situations. Indeed, MI can be used by pediatric clinicians and met with discord, ambivalence, or disinterest. In some situations, it is possible that discord or "resistance" from patients is due to having different values or goals than the clinician. With this in mind, it is critical for pediatric clinicians to engage in continued self-reflection and awareness of the broader spectrum of systems, community, family, and individual-based factors influencing patients and themselves, respectively. Instead of behavior change always being the goal (eg, seeking out mental health support), pediatric clinicians are encouraged to consider *continued partnership* as a goal (eg, demonstrating that you are ready and willing to talk about mental health supports when a family is interested). Certainly, the longitudinal relationships in primary care medicine in particular lend themselves to having discussions about behavior change over time and not attempting to solve challenges in a single visit.

Application to Behavioral and Mental Health

Pediatric clinicians in primary care are often the first line for the assessment and management of behavioral and mental health concerns.[9] In fact, the American Academy of Pediatrics recommends that pediatric clinicians deliver behavioral health care.[10] Concerns can be brought to pediatric clinicians by the patient and family; opportunities for concerns to be identified exist during both routine well checks or acute care visits.[11] In either case, the MI spirit and core communication skills can help evoke richer data to facilitate assessment/disposition, treatment planning, and an understanding of readiness to change. Further, MI affords pediatric clinicians a pathway for engagement around mental health concerns that walks the line between overly normalizing patient/family concerns that can lead to invalidation and overpathologization of symptoms.

MI communication skills (OARS) can be used to demonstrate that the pediatric clinician understands the patient/family experience and to provide support to families about concerning symptoms. Naming specific positive behaviors or affirming positive acts can be useful to highlight strengths that the patient/family possess and to encourage movement in positive directions. This can be particularly impactful as it applies to mental health or behavioral health changes in behavior as often families feel a large external locus of control related to change. Further, using OARS within the spirit of MI is inherently reinforcing to families in the context of trust building and validation, thus increasing the likelihood that they will get the treatment that they both want and is indicated. Additionally, pediatric clinicians practicing MI are called to allow for the goals in patient interactions to shift from behavior change to ongoing partnerships. This approach that is attuned to patient and family motivation and experience makes possible an ongoing dialog in cases in which families/patients present resistance around concerns a medical team may have related to mental health.

Stigma regarding mental health concerns is an ever-present shadow that can impede assessment and treatment of symptoms. There is clear evidence that stigma around mental health decreases help-seeking behaviors.[12] MI's evocative nature requires the pediatric clinician to focus attention on the patient/family concerns and reasons for change. The intention to fully understand what a patient/family values can shift attention away from "symptoms" and move toward understanding how the symptoms are impacting values and goals. This shift away from symptoms or diagnoses can reduce stigma by focusing on helping the patient/family get closer to the life they want to lead.

Finally, pediatric clinicians often report less comfort providing interventions for mental or behavioral health concerns as compared to their comfort with assessment or referral.[13] With this in mind, MI represents a valuable approach as it is an intervention in and of itself. Notably, it is unlikely to be the only intervention required to treat a mental health concern, but it is germane to many evidence-based mental health treatments. Thus, pediatric clinicians can be reassured that by integrating MI into their practice they are actively providing an intervention for presenting mental or behavioral health concerns.

CASE STUDIES: HOW CAN YOU USE MOTIVATIONAL INTERVIEWING FOR MENTAL AND BEHAVIORAL HEALTH CONCERNS IN PRIMARY CARE?

MI is a promising intervention strategy for pediatric clinicians, and mastery of MI requires continued practice. Novice learners of MI are recommended to begin with practicing demonstration of the MI spirit,[14] which requires self-reflection, awareness of personal biases, and willingness to partner with the person and family in a nonjudgmental way. The following case studies were constructed to support active learning through application of the foundational knowledge of MI to cases with mental and behavioral health concerns. We invite readers to walk through the cases as a strategy to promote skill development for learning the tasks of MI (**Table 2**) and to identify potential pitfalls and mitigation strategies when deploying MI (**Table 3**).

Continuing Motivational Interviewing Education

Although there is not a standard amount of training to demonstrate proficiency, Miller and Rollnick[1] recommend repeated practice of MI skills and spirit to promote learning. If possible, supervision by those trained in MI, such as those in the Motivational Interviewing Network of Trainers (MINT), can help provide targeted feedback and growth. Educational applications and use of artificial intelligence technology[15,16] also provide promising avenues for MI training. In order to promote continued learning, pediatric clinicians may find it helpful to practice outside of patient interactions and may choose to role play common clinical scenarios with colleagues. For skill building and reflection, pediatric clinicians may also choose to listen to audio recordings of themselves in practice with written permission from patients. The MINT Web site (https://

Table 2
Case study: progression through the tasks of motivational interviewing when discussing mental health in pediatrics

You are seeing a 5 year old male individual, Zaden, for a concern about poor sleep for the past month. His teachers have expressed concerned that Zaden is irritable and poorly focused during the school day. He has been staying up until 1 AM looking at his tablet and needs to wake up at 6 AM to get ready for school. His mother, Stephanie, who sleeps poorly herself, is concerned about his school performance. She alludes to a family history of bipolar disorder and is wondering if this could be a sign of a mental health issue for her son. For the past week, Zaden has been asking his mother if he can stay home from kindergarten due to these symptoms, which prompted today's visit		
Tasks of MI	*Sample Dialog*	*Tips for Task*
Engaging: building trust and rapport	*What are your concerns about Zaden?* *Tell me more about what is worrying you*	You may "only" get to the point of engagement in an encounter—that is okay! Engaging is critical and can help encourage and enrich future conversations
Stephanie: "My son is not *sleeping. I am really concerned that something is wrong. My aunt used to stay up for these long stretches, and they said she was bipolar. I just don't know what to do."*		
Focusing: agreeing on where to center the conversation with the patient/caregiver	*You're concerned about where some of the sleep troubles may be coming from. This could be caused by several different things. Would you be willing to tell me more about his sleep routines?*	Finding a place to focus is artful. When focusing, ask yourself: Did I allow the patient to choose the topic rather than choosing it myself? Am I still aligning with the family's values?
Stephanie: "We usually get home around 5:30. By the time I get dinner done and he takes a bath, it is close to 8:30. I usually give him the tablet in his room to help him get to sleep, and then I try to clean up or do a few things for myself. It is so hard to get a break these days. I'll wake up and notice he is still on that tablet after I've gone to sleep."		
Evoking: allowing space for the patient/caregiver to think about change aloud and talk about reasons for change in the context of their lived experiences	*Evenings can be really busy and challenging. If you had time, what parts of the routine do you think are most important to shift?*	Evoking may inspire many responses, including "Change talk" (*I really want him to have a consistent bedtime.*) and/or "Sustain talk" (*It might be too hard.*) Don't shy away from sustain talk— affirm and explore ambivalence about family-centered goal about sleep

(*continued on next page*)

Table 2
(continued)

Stephanie: "I really want him to have a consistent bedtime. It might be time to do something about the tablet, I don't know. It might be too hard. But I don't think he is getting enough sleep overall, and I want him to get the most out of kindergarten."		
Planning: clarifying the specifics of change alongside the patient/caregiver	*"How ready do you feel to make some adjustments to the bedtime routine, on a scale of 1 (not at all ready) to 10 (ready to start immediately)?"* *"How can I be most helpful in supporting your goals?"*	When the patient is ready, make a specific and measurable plan Beware of the "fixing reflex" and the urge to make a change plan before the patient is ready
Stephanie: "I feel ready, maybe a 7. I'm scared it won't work and he will get upset with me. And I am already tired at the end of the day. I think I need help knowing how to keep him calm because he's so used to falling asleep watching the tablet."		
Summary: At this point in the encounter, you have identified concerns, goals, and barriers from Zaden's mom. Like many presenting concerns in the pediatric setting, there is complexity and nuance here; the spirit of MI can help to navigate these. The end-point for each individual encounter may vary—for this encounter, the endpoint may be engaging Stephanie in strategies to decrease Zaden's screen time and offer her techniques to manage his response when the tablet is removed. There may be encounters where MI techniques are employed and the visit accomplishes establishing trust, rapport, and a foundation for future visits. Pediatric clinicians are the guides and should allow patient and family readiness to lead conversations about health optimization and behavior change		

Table 3
Case study: using motivational interviewing in pediatrics to navigate conversations about mental health

You are in primary care clinic seeing a 14 year old female individual, Jackie, who is there for her yearly physical. She is joined by her mother, Janelle. Jackie completes a Patient Health Questionnaire (PHQ-9) screening measure, and her answers are concerning for depressive symptoms. After reviewing Jackie's history, obtaining some basic information and building an initial rapport, you discuss the screening results and concern for depression. Jackie appears a bit sullen. Her mother is dismissive of the screener's validity and says, "Oh, she's fine." You acknowledge that you agree she's doing well overall and express curiosity as to whether she could optimize her well-being with some mental health support

Potential Pitfalls	*MI Approach*	*Sample Dialog (skill)*
Clinician might feel an urge to "fix" this situation when the screener results	In order to demonstrate that patient and family members are collaborators in care, use open-ended questions for additional information gathering before making a plan	*"Janelle, What are your reactions to the results of this screening?"* *"Jackie, what do you think about these screening results?"* (open question) *"What changes have you noticed with Jackie over the past year?"* *"What changes have you noticed in yourself over the past year?"* (open question)
Pediatric clinician may feel an urge to defend the test's validity	Use reflection to show that you appreciate the concern Ask permission to focus the conversation further Use ask-offer-ask to provide information and encourage further reflection and discussion	*"You're concerned that the screening isn't showing what you see in Jackie's everyday life."* (reflection). *"Would it be ok with you if we take a minute to talk about the purpose of the screening?"* (asking permission) *"What are your thoughts about this screener and why we ask people to complete it?"* (ask) *"Yes, it does ask about people's mood. Would it be ok if I add to that information?"* *"The screener that you completed today is meant to start a conversation. Although you are thinking it is inaccurate, the hope is that we can talk more about what is really happening and how to help Jackie."* (offer) *"How does that sound to you?"* (ask)

(*continued on next page*)

Table 3
(continued)

Frustration arises at the end of visit when there is not a "resolution"	Use a summary to highlight what was discussed at the visit. Name specific short-term goals that can help with attainment of the long-term goal Use an open-ended question to honor the family's current readiness to change and create openness to continue to discuss change in the future	*"It's been so valuable today to hear about Jackie's goals and your hopes for her. Although you were unsure about the screening results initially, you are committed to helping her feel better. You're not currently interested in therapy referrals. As an immediate next step, you plan to schedule a meeting with the school counselor on Monday to talk more about treatment options."* (summarizing) *"What would be the best way for us to stay in contact in case additional support is needed?"* (open-ended question)

motivationalinterviewing.org/) is a helpful resource for up-to-date training materials, research, and learning opportunities.

SUMMARY

This article presented the core components of MI, the inherent cultural responsiveness of MI, and therefore the broad applicability of MI to concerns in primary care, especially regarding mental and behavioral health. The case studies provided an opportunity for active learning and application of MI skills in a culturally-responsive manner. Although we recognize that amplifying the inherent culturally-responsive aspects of MI may feel novel for pediatric clinicians, we emphasize that this is key to effective use of MI with mental and behavioral health concerns, given the associated barriers, hesitations, and complexity. MI is uniquely positioned to support the pediatric clinicians in navigating mental health discussions in a compassionate, strengths-promoting partnership with patients and caregivers.

MI offers an effective, culturally-responsive approach to mental and behavioral health. As pediatric clinicians enhance their MI skillset, MI becomes a "way of being" that permeates into all aspects of their clinical practice. This increases the likelihood that their clinical practice will not only be more impactful to patients and families but also more rewarding as these relationships deepen. This transformation of practice requires ongoing self-reflection, whereby pediatric clinicians increase the awareness of their own values and biases. This conscious awareness enables the cultivation of a nonjudgmental approach and space to explore and understand the different perspectives, experiences, and values of patients that the pediatric clinician can use to strengthen motivation to engage in a shared goal. Finally, the values of autonomy, patient strengths, and empowerment align with core tenants of pediatric primary care practice and translated into action by the pediatric clinician using MI to promote and address mental and behavioral health.

CLINICS CARE POINTS

A variety of barriers exist that can make doing MI challenging. These practical approaches to troubleshooting can help.

- Short windows of time available for interactions.
  - MI skills can be deployed even when time is short, as a part of routine practice. Resisting the urge to speed through and using open-ended questions is the best use of your time when behavior change is the goal.
- Patients or family members may express resistance toward change.
  - Avoid trying to persuade; honor and accept the person's readiness to change.
- Clinical environment includes learners (students, residents, and so forth).
  - Create safe learning spaces; role play with MI language and/or model MI during direct observation.
- Emergency occurs during visit.
  - Priorities can be shifted during visit to best accommodate patients' safety and needs.
- Discordance between family's priorities and pediatric clinician's priorities.
  - Resist the "fixing reflex" or need to "fix" or resolve a concern immediately.
- Lots of anticipatory guidance needs to be provided during visit.
  - Prioritize using MI for a shared agenda item and provide brief standard anticipatory guidance for topics that are not identified as a shared goal with the family.

DISCLOSURE

The authors have nothing to disclose.

REFERENCES

1. Miller WR, Rollnick S. Motivational interviewing: helping people change and grow. New York, NY: Guilford Publications; 2023.
2. Lundahl B, Burke BL. The effectiveness and applicability of motivational interviewing: a practice-friendly review of four meta-analyses. J Clin Psychol 2009; 65(11):1232–45.
3. DiClemente CC, Corno CM, Graydon MM, et al. Motivational interviewing, enhancement, and brief interventions over the last decade: A review of reviews of efficacy and effectiveness. Psychol Addict Behav 2017;31(8):862–87.
4. Morton K, Beauchamp M, Prothero A, et al. The effectiveness of motivational interviewing for health behaviour change in primary care settings: a systematic review. Health Psychol Rev 2015;9(2):205–23.
5. Miller WRR. Motivational interviewing: helping people change. 3rd edition. New York, NY: The Guilford Press; 2013.
6. Rogers CR. A way of being. Boston, MA: Houghton Mifflin; 1980.
7. Lopez SJ, Snyder CR. Oxford handbook of positive psychology. Oxford library of psychology. 2nd edition. Oxford University Press Oxford; 2011.
8. Physicians AAoF. Primary Care. 2024. Available at: https://www.aafp.org/about/policies/all/primary-care.html. [Accessed 1 February 2024].
9. O'Brien D, Harvey K, Howse J, et al. Barriers to managing child and adolescent mental health problems: a systematic review of primary care practitioners' perceptions. Br J Gen Pract 2016;66(651):e693–707.
10. Committee on Psychosocial Aspects of C, Family H, Task Force on Mental H. Policy statement–The future of pediatrics: mental health competencies for pediatric primary care. Pediatrics 2009;124(1):410–21.
11. Brino KAS. Pediatric Mental Health and the Power of Primary Care: Practical Approaches and Validating Challenges. J Pediatr Health Care 2020;34(2):e12–20.
12. Schnyder N, Panczak R, Groth N, et al. Association between mental health-related stigma and active help-seeking: systematic review and meta-analysis. Br J Psychiatry 2017;210(4):261–8.
13. Bettencourt AF, Ferro RA, Williams JL, et al. Pediatric Primary Care Provider Comfort with Mental Health Practices: A Needs Assessment of Regions with Shortages of Treatment Access. Acad Psychiatry 2021;45(4):429–34.
14. Miller WR, Moyers TB. Eight Stages in Learning Motivational Interviewing. J Teach Addict 2006/01/01 2006;5(1):3–17.
15. Vasoya MM, Shivakumar A, Pappu S, et al. ReadMI: An Innovative App to Support Training in Motivational Interviewing. Journal of Graduate Medical Education 2019;11(3):344–6.
16. Hershberger PJ, Pei Y, Bricker DA, et al. Advancing Motivational Interviewing Training with Artificial Intelligence: ReadMI. Adv Med Educ Pract 2021/06/04 2021;12(null):613–8.

Practice-Based Models of Pediatric Mental Health Care

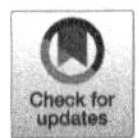

Chuan Mei Lee, MD, MA[a,b,*], Jayme Congdon, MD, MS[c,d], Christina Joy, MD[e], Barry Sarvet, MD[f]

KEYWORDS

- Integrated behavioral health • Pediatrics • Primary care
- Child psychiatry access program • Primary care behavioral health
- Collaborative care model

KEY POINTS

- As many as 20% of all children and adolescents have an identified mental health condition annually, but only about 10% of youth receive mental health services.
- Coronavirus disease 2019 pandemic has only exacerbated these concerns, with studies showing significant increases in depression and anxiety symptoms globally.
- There is no one-size-fits-all model of integrating behavioral health services in pediatric primary care settings, and models vary in scope and strategies for implementation.

INTRODUCTION

Behavioral health disorders among children and adolescents in the United States (US) are common yet undertreated. As many as 20% of all children and adolescents have an identified mental health condition annually, but only about 10% of youth receive mental health services.[1] The coronavirus disease 2019 (COVID-19) pandemic has only exacerbated these concerns, with studies showing significant increases in depression and anxiety symptoms globally.[2] In 2021, the American Academy of Pediatrics (AAP), the American Academy of Child and Adolescent Psychiatry (AACAP), and the Children's Hospital Association jointly declared a national emergency in child and adolescent mental health,[3] and the US Surgeon General issued a public health advisory on youth mental health, calling for urgent action.[4]

[a] Department of Psychiatry and Behavioral Sciences, UCSF, 675 18th Street, Box 3132, San Francisco, CA 94143, USA; [b] Clinical Excellence Research Center, Stanford University School of Medicine, Stanford, CA, USA; [c] Department of Pediatrics, UCSF, 675 18th Street, Box 3132, San Francisco, CA 94143, USA; [d] Philip R. Lee Institute for Health Policy Studies, UCSF, San Francisco, CA, USA; [e] Department of Child and Adolescent Psychiatry and Behavioral Sciences, Children's Hospital of Philadelphia, Hub for Clinical Collaboration, DCAPBS, 3500 Civic Center Boulevard, 12th floor, Philadelphia, PA 19104, USA; [f] Department of Psychiatry, University of Massachusetts Medical School – Baystate, 759 Chestnut Street, WG703, Springfield, MA 01199, USA
* Corresponding author.
E-mail address: chuanmei.lee@ucsf.edu

Pediatr Clin N Am 71 (2024) 1059–1071
https://doi.org/10.1016/j.pcl.2024.07.013 **pediatric.theclinics.com**

However, there are not enough specialty mental health providers to meet this growing need for youth mental health services. Longstanding workforce shortages of child and adolescent psychiatrists[5] have translated into long wait times for child psychiatry appointments.[6] A cross-sectional study of US youth suicides found an association between youth suicide rates and county mental health professional workforce shortages, even after adjusting for county demographic and socioeconomic characteristics, suggesting the importance of an adequate workforce to meet youth behavioral health needs.[7]

Pediatric primary care is uniquely positioned to address youth behavioral health needs as it is widely accessible to children and adolescents. Over 90% of youth have seen a primary care provider (PCP) in the past 12 months.[8] Often PCPs have a longitudinal relationship with children and families and are frequently the first point of contact to discuss behavioral health concerns. Therefore, over the past decade, both the AAP and AACAP have called upon PCPs to deliver behavioral health services in pediatric primary care settings.[9,10]

However, there is no one-size-fits-all model of integrating behavioral health services in pediatric primary care settings, and models vary in scope and strategies for implementation.[11] This article describes 3 common pediatric models of integrated care: (1) the Child Psychiatry Access Program (CPAP) model, (2) the Primary Care Behavioral Health (PCBH) model, and (3) the Collaborative Care Model (CoCM). We compare the 3 models and summarize their key features.

CHILD PSYCHIATRY ACCESS PROGRAM

CPAPs, also known as Pediatric Mental Health Care Access Programs, are centralized (often statewide) programs that offer free, remote pediatric mental health consultation services, care coordination with referrals to local mental health care resources, and continuing mental health education for pediatric PCPs.[12] These programs support PCPs and other pediatric frontline clinicians (eg, school-based clinicians, emergency department physicians) in addressing child and adolescent mental health needs and improving access to pediatric mental health care in general medical settings. PCPs can call a mental health specialist in real-time and receive answers to their consultation questions, in an interaction that is meant to be both educational and practical. *Case 1* shows an example of a consultation call with a CPAP child psychiatry consultant.

Since the first statewide CPAP—Massachusetts Child Psychiatry Access Project—pioneered this approach 20 years ago, [13] this practice-based model has spread to almost all states in the US.[14] Recent expansions have been supported by waves of federal grant funding from the Health Resources and Services Administration (HRSA).[15] Most CPAPs are funded by a combination of state and federal government funding, as well as philanthropy, though without a formal payment model, long-term financial sustainability remains uncertain for many programs.[16]

Despite the significant federal investment and expansion of CPAPs, evidence to support the effectiveness of consultation mostly comes from the adult literature.[17] Systematic reviews focused on CPAPs have found that most studies are descriptive, commonly reporting program adoption and/or provider experience outcomes.[12,18,19] This underscores the need for more research that examines patient-level mental health outcomes, though this has been challenging given that, for the most part, CPAPs are provider-level interventions.[12] Furthermore, having a standardized set of program criteria and outcomes would help facilitate comparisons across different programs.[20]

CASE 1

Dr Singh is a pediatrician practicing in rural California. This morning she saw Cy, a 17 year-old non-binary teen struggling with depression and anxiety since their mother's death a year ago. Dr Singh had started Cy on fluoxetine 10 mg daily, increased it to 20 mg daily about a month ago, and had been trying to help the teen find a therapist through their insurance network to no avail. However, Cy reported worsening anxiety after starting fluoxetine, and Dr Singh was unsure of next steps. She decided to call the California CPAP warmline[21] for consultation during her lunch break.

Dr Kim, a child and adolescent psychiatrist, answered the telephone call. As he listened to Dr Singh's case, he asked if the patient had completed any mental health measures. Because Dr Singh had called the CPAP before and had attended several CPAP-sponsored webinars, she had already obtained Patient Health Questionnaire-9 (PHQ-9) and General Anxiety Disorder-7 (GAD-7) measures. Cy had a PHQ-9 score of 10 with no suicidality and a worsening GAD-7 score of 18. With this information, Dr Kim recommended that Dr Singh continue to increase the fluoxetine by 10 mg increments every 3 to 4 weeks with follow up (to a maximum dose of 60 mg daily) until symptoms are sufficiently improved, noting that often anxiety symptoms may require a higher dose of fluoxetine for a response. Dr Kim also noted that if the patient experiences no improvement after 2 months, the PCP should consider switching to another selective serotonin reuptake inhibitor medication.

Dr Kim then asked the PCP if she wanted her call to be transferred to a licensed clinical social worker for therapy referrals in Cy's community. Dr Singh stated that while she did not have time today to stay on the phone, she would schedule another time to speak with the social worker for resource referrals. Dr Kim also mentioned to Dr Singh that she would sign up for a webinar on anxiety disorders on the CPAP's website.

PRIMARY CARE BEHAVIORAL HEALTH

PCBH is a team-based model with behavioral health clinicians, such as social workers, counselors, therapists, or psychologists, embedded in a primary care setting.[22] In a clinic employing a PCBH model, PCPs perform the initial screening and identification of patients who may benefit from additional behavioral health support. Primary care-based behavioral health clinicians may become involved in a patient's care due to behavioral health symptoms or to address psychosocial factors influencing other health outcomes or health behaviors. Commonly, behavioral health team members provide triage and response to positive behavioral health screens, secondary screening and assessment, brief interventions, psychosocial therapy, and referrals to specialty behavioral health services. In some cases, a behavioral health clinician may not directly interface with patients, instead providing brief consultation and guidance to the PCP. The PCBH model typically prioritizes assessing and intervening within the primary care setting initially, reserving referrals to specialty behavioral health care for patients with persistent or severe symptoms or impairment. When specialty behavioral health care is indicated, the behavioral health clinician serves as a liaison and provides warm handoffs to specialty providers. PCBH can also act as a bridge when there are delays in receiving specialty services. *Case 2* illustrates a common workflow within a primary care clinic employing a PCBH model.

There is evidence to support PCBH across the "quadruple aim" of health care (ie, patient experience, health outcomes, provider outcomes, and cost).[23] Behavioral health integration (BHI) has been shown to improve primary care engagement,[24] increased access to behavioral health services,[25] and patient satisfaction.[26] PCBH also has the potential to promote health equity, with some studies demonstrating disproportionate benefit for children from marginalized racial and ethnic groups.[27,28] In a meta-analysis of randomized controlled trials, health outcomes were better with integrated behavioral health compared to usual primary care.[29] A real-world implementation of PCBH across a large network of primary care clinics in Massachusetts provides additional evidence of the benefits of PCBH to patients' access and quality of care, and additionally demonstrated that participating providers had greater self-efficacy, satisfaction, and confidence in managing mild to moderate behavioral health problems.[30] The Massachusetts example illustrates how integrating behavioral health clinicians not only support provider experience, but also has the potential to develop behavioral health competencies across the health care team,[31] which is a known barrier to identifying and managing behavioral health problems in pediatric primary care.[32]

Despite the benefits of PCBH, there remain barriers to its implementation. The available behavioral health workforce, again, falls far short of the demand.[33] One component of this workforce shortage is some degree of misalignment between the training of behavioral health clinicians and their potential role within a PCBH model, necessitating efforts to prepare and attract individuals for primary care-based roles.[33] Financing has also been raised as a barrier to implementing and sustaining PCBH.[34] For example, traditional fee-for-service arrangements have prevented integrated clinics from obtaining reimbursement for co-located behavioral health services provided on the same day as a medical visit. Additionally, mental health carve-outs that limit reimbursement to a specified network of behavioral health providers or organizations have prevented reimbursement of the primary care-based behavioral health clinicians. However, the feasibility of PCBH has improved with recent payment reforms that address these barriers and facilitate health system integration (eg, Affordable Care Act, Mental Health Parity and Addiction Equity Act, and Medicaid expansion).[34] Future studies are needed to evaluate the cost and sustainability of PCBH implementation in the wake of these reforms. Such work would build on the few existing studies linking PCBH to more optimal health care utilization, such as fewer preventable hospitalizations, fewer referrals to specialty mental health, and higher revenue generation.[26,35,36]

CASE 2

Ana is a pediatric nurse practitioner seeing Jess, a 12-year-old girl presenting to an acute primary care visit for episodes of shortness of breath. After completing a focused history and physical examination, Ana suspects that Jess is having panic attacks that started in the context of a recent conflict at school. With permission from Jess and her mother, Ana steps out to touch base with the clinic's licensed clinical social worker, Lea. Lea has another patient to see first, but if the family can wait, she has time to check in with Ana. Lea suggests that Jess complete a PHQ-9 and GAD-7 while she waits.

After about 15 min, Lea meets Jess and her mother. They spend more time discussing her symptoms, recent stressors, strengths and sources of support, and other social drivers of health. Lea offers support and suggests self-management techniques for coping with stress and anxiety. Based on their conversation, and the PHQ-9 and GAD-7 results, Lea finds that Jess has a mild presentation of panic disorder. Given the context of good social support, she recommends brief psychotherapy for the initial treatment plan and arranges to follow-up by phone the following week. Lea describes the encounter and plan in a brief note in the electronic medical record, which she shares with Ana and Jess's PCP.

COLLABORATIVE CARE MODEL

The CoCM is an evidence-based model for integrating primary care and behavioral health treatment, demonstrating improved patient outcomes, team collaboration, and provider and patient satisfaction in primary care settings.[37,38] The CoCM team consists of a PCP, a behavioral health care manager (BHCM), and a psychiatric consultant. Once a patient with behavioral concerns is identified (through routine screening or their presentation to care), the PCP connects the patient and family to the BHCM. The BHCM, who is generally based in the primary care clinic, provides structured initial and follow-up assessments, basic psychoeducation and self-management skills, as well as brief, evidenced-based psychotherapeutic interventions.[39] The BHCM works closely with the PCP and helps manage a caseload of patients using a patient registry.

The patient registry is an important element in the implementation and operation of the CoCM, enabling team members to keep track of identified patients, monitor progress over time, and prioritize care. The registry includes patient information, treatment status, key service dates (eg, first and most recent visits with the BHCM, most recent psychiatric case review, number of weeks spent in treatment, and upcoming appointments), clinical progress with measurement-based tools (eg, the PHQ-9 for depression), interventions being utilized (eg, psychotherapy and/or medications), and flags for safety risk or discussion at next psychiatric case review.[39]

The psychiatric consultant, who is often located off-site, and BHCM have weekly meetings, where new patients are presented, and patients who are not improving are discussed. The psychiatric consultant advises the team on each patient in the registry and makes recommendations regarding diagnoses and treatments, which are then relayed to the PCP for implementation. The psychiatric consultant is also available to the PCP for consultation as needed.[39] In this way, patients with mild to moderate symptoms are managed by the PCP until treatment targets are achieved, while those with severe or chronic symptoms are linked for referral to specialty mental health care by the BHCM. Only a handful of patients (eg, challenging patients or those who have not been served by indirect consultation) are directly evaluated by the psychiatric consultant. *Case 3* illustrates an example of a young child's treatment within a clinic utilizing the CoCM.

The CoCM has been shown to be effective in improving behavioral health outcomes among pediatric populations in multiple randomized controlled trials.[29] At its core, CoCM is a population health model that targets a whole population of patients under a PCP's care and not just those who present with mental health concerns in a waiting room, providing populations with better access to quality mental health care.[39] CoCM supports measurement-based "treatment to target" by using validated and standardized patient measures to routinely monitor a patient's progress and treatments adjusted until clinical goals are reached. Evidenced-based brief psychotherapies are offered to patients, and all of the team are accountable for the care delivered.[39] Identifying and treating patients with mental health concerns proactively prevents progression and associated comorbidities, as well as the utilization of more intensive services.[38,40]

Some challenges to CoCM implementation include the complexity of this multicomponent model and the practice change required to carry it out. Team members may need to learn unfamiliar ways of practice to carry out their role within the model, including new workflows to accommodate using measurement-based care, a patient registry, evidence-based treatments, and coordination among different team members. It can be overwhelming for a BHCM to provide brief psychotherapy, manage the registry, do outreach, and coordinate outside referrals to specialists and other psychosocial supports. Financial feasibility remains an issue as there is a large upfront cost to setting up the model. While the Centers for Medicaid and Medicare Services has introduced a set of bundled Current Procedural Terminology (CPT) codes to reimburse CoCM activities, the funding is often insufficient and confusing to navigate for providers.[40]

CASE 3

Zoe is a 5-year-old girl presenting for her annual well-child visit. As a part of the annual visit, Zoe's mom fills out the Pediatric Symptom Checklist. Her pediatrician, Dr Garcia, reviews the screening tool and notes a significantly elevated score on the attention subscale. On further probing, Zoe's mom shares that Zoe struggles with intense behavioral outbursts at home and problems focusing in school. Her teacher has remarked that compared to her peers, Zoe has a difficult time settling down after recess, staying in her seat, and waiting for her turn.

Dr Garcia finds Adam, a BHCM, in the clinic, and he is available to do a "warm handoff," where the family is able to meet Adam and schedule a visit with him to further assess Zoe's symptoms.

Subsequently, Adam does a thorough evaluation and has Zoe's mom and teacher complete Vanderbilt Assessment Scales for attention deficit hyperactivity disorder (ADHD) that confirm his initial clinical impressions. During their weekly case review meeting, the psychiatric consultant, Dr Marcus, agrees with Adam's provisional diagnosis of ADHD, and together they come up with a treatment plan.

Adam discusses the diagnosis and treatment plan with Zoe's mom and Dr Garcia. Zoe's mom is hesitant about starting medications given Zoe's age and expresses desire to pursue an evidence-based behavior therapy, which Adam initiates. The family is followed regularly, with the help of a registry, and consultation is provided by Dr Marcus as needed.

After several months, Adam repeats the Vanderbilt Assessment Scales, and Zoe's scores are largely unchanged. Zoe and her mom have been coming to all their appointments, and Zoe's mom has been implementing behavioral strategies as suggested by Adam at home. Since there is minimal improvement in Zoe's ADHD symptoms with behavior therapy, the case was reviewed again with Dr Marcus during their weekly meeting. Given Zoe's continued struggles at home and school, Dr Marcus discusses the option of starting a stimulant medication to target her symptoms. In the next session with Zoe's mom, Adam discusses the Vanderbilt Assessment Scale results and ascertains any concerns about starting medication. Dr Marcus provides education to Adam about the benefits of ADHD treatment with stimulants, disadvantages of not adequately treating ADHD, and potential side effects of stimulant medication. Adam takes this information and shares it with the family. He also offers the family opportunity to discuss concerns further directly with Dr Marcus. Mom feels more empowered to try a stimulant medication with Zoe.

Adam informs Dr Garcia of the change in the treatment plan and the family's wish for a trial of a stimulant medication. Dr Marcus reaches out to Dr Garcia to discuss initial reasonable medication choices, how to initiate and titrate stimulants, and their side effects. Dr Garcia decides to prescribe methylphenidate and feels confident managing the stimulant knowing that Dr Marcus is readily available for questions.

DISCUSSION

Given the significant variation in the implementation of each of the 3 models of BHI in pediatric primary care settings described earlier, it is difficult to differentiate them precisely. Each model employs similar principles and tactics such as cultivating collaborative interprofessional relationships, deploying evidence-based treatment, providing interprofessional and direct clinical consultation, and care coordination. It is also notable that the models are not mutually exclusive. As an example, a primary care practice utilizing the PCBH model with an embedded behavioral health clinician may operate in a region covered by a CPAP and utilize the CPAP for psychiatric consultation. In another example, a primary care practice may utilize the CoCM for a subset of patients in the practice panel with a specific diagnosis (ie, adolescent depression) while employing the PCBH model for general behavioral health needs arising from the panel.

A common framework from the Substance Abuse and Mental Health Services Administration (SAMHSA) and the HRSA proposes 6 levels of integration, ranging from coordinated care to co-located care to integrated care (**Fig. 1**).[41] In this framework, coordinated care refers to communication and coordination of care between behavioral health and primary care; co-located care designates closer collaboration due to physical proximity in the same practice space; and integrated care indicates practice change that merges behavioral health and primary care.

One of the limitations of the SAMHSA-HRSA framework, which has become increasingly apparent since the COVID-19 pandemic is the primacy of physical adjacency as a defining characteristic for situating programs within a hierarchical ("levels") framework. Specifically, with the advent of telehealth, providers have discovered that rich collaborative relationships can develop over large distances, and that physical proximity is not necessary for even the highest levels of integration. For example, in the CPAP model, it is possible for highly engaged psychiatric consultants to develop highly integrated relationships with practices without ever meeting anyone in the practice in person. In these instances, the CPAP consultants become unofficial members of the primary care team by virtue of talking with members of the practice frequently and even providing longitudinal follow-up consultation on challenging patients. Conversely, it has been quite apparent that physical proximity alone or co-location does not ensure any meaningful integration. For example, authors have observed practice settings including behavioral health providers who interact minimally with the rest of the pediatric team. This is often due to practice management policies in which the behavioral health providers are expected to maximize billable activity, resulting in limited availability for engaging new patients or interacting with members of the primary care team.

Table 1 summarizes key characteristics of the 3 models. While all models necessitate and promote changes in clinical workflow in the pediatric primary care practice and the introduction of new roles within the immediate and/or extended primary care team, each of these 3 models have distinctly different emphases and priorities, as described in the following sections.

Direct Provision of Psychotherapy Versus Referring Out

One of the core principles in the CoCM is termed "measurement-based treatment to target." This not only refers to the included feature of measurement-based care in the model, but also to the fact that patients are routinely receiving evidence-based psychotherapeutic intervention in the primary care practice setting. While PCBH includes brief psychotherapy provided by the embedded behavioral health clinician for selected patients, there is often more of an emphasis on referrals to behavioral health clinicians external to the practice and coordinating this external treatment within the patient's overall treatment plan. Practices working with CPAPs may or may not have internal resources to provide psychotherapy and regardless of this, psychotherapy treatment

COORDINATED KEY ELEMENT: COMMUNICATION		CO-LOCATED KEY ELEMENT: PHYSICAL PROXIMITY		INTEGRATED KEY ELEMENT: PRACTICE CHANGE	
LEVEL 1 Minimal Collaboration	LEVEL 2 Basic Collaboration at a Distance	LEVEL 3 Basic Collaboration Onsite	LEVEL 4 Close Collaboration Onsite with Some System Integration	LEVEL 5 Close Collaboration Approaching an Integrated Practice	LEVEL 6 Full Collaboration in a Transformed/ Merged Integrated Practice
Behavioral health, primary care and other healthcare providers work:					
In separate facilities, where they:	In separate facilities, where they:	In same facility not necessarily same offices, where they:	In same space within the same facility, where they:	In same space within the same facility (some shared space), where they:	In same space within the same facility, sharing all practice space, where they:
▸▸ Have separate systems ▸▸ Communicate about cases only rarely and under compelling circumstances ▸▸ Communicate, driven by provider need ▸▸ May never meet in person ▸▸ Have limited understanding of each other's roles	▸▸ Have separate systems ▸▸ Communicate periodically about shared patients ▸▸ Communicate, driven by specific patient issues ▸▸ May meet as part of larger community ▸▸ Appreciate each other's roles as resources	▸▸ Have separate systems ▸▸ Communicate regularly about shared patients, by phone or e-mail ▸▸ Collaborate, driven by need for each other's services and more reliable referral ▸▸ Meet occasionally to discuss cases due to close proximity ▸▸ Feel part of a larger yet non-formal team	▸▸ Share some systems, like scheduling or medical records ▸▸ Communicate in person as needed ▸▸ Collaborate, driven by need for consultation and coordinated plans for difficult patients ▸▸ Have regular face-to-face interactions about some patients ▸▸ Have a basic understanding of roles and culture	▸▸ Actively seek system solutions together or develop work-a-rounds ▸▸ Communicate frequently in person ▸▸ Collaborate, driven by desire to be a member of the care team ▸▸ Have regular team meetings to discuss overall patient care and specific patient issues ▸▸ Have an in-depth understanding of roles and culture	▸▸ Have resolved most or all system issues, functioning as one integrated system ▸▸ Communicate consistently at the system, team and individual levels ▸▸ Collaborate, driven by shared concept of team care ▸▸ Have formal and informal meetings to support integrated model of care ▸▸ Have roles and cultures that blur or blend

Fig. 1. The Substance Abuse and Mental Health Services Administration-Health Resources and Services Administration framework (SAMHSA-HRSA)

Table 1
Behavioral Health Integration (BHI) models in pediatric clinical settings compared

Program Characteristic	CPAP	PCBH	CoCM
Relationships			
BH provider full member of primary care team	2	5	5
BH provider is an external resource accessible to primary care team	5	1	1
Timing of BH involvement			
BH provider available in real time to respond to clinical needs when they present in practice	4	5	5
BH provider involvement and collaboration is scheduled for later	5	5	5
BH role is reactive or "on demand"	5	5	5
BH role is proactive (offered before someone asks for help)[a]	3	4	5
Documentation of BH services			
In-shared record	2	5	5
Location of BH services			
In primary care practice suite	2	5	5
BH services offered			
Interprofessional consultation			
By integrated behavioral health clinician	3	5	5
By child and adolescent psychiatrist	5	2	5
Direct patient assessment			
By integrated behavioral health clinician	3	5	5
By child and adolescent psychiatrist	4	2	4
Care coordination/Resource navigation-information to practice	5	5	5
Care coordination/Resource navigation-warm hand-offs	3	5	5
Psychotherapy provided directly	2	4	5
Population health features			
Systematic screening	3	4	5
Measurement-based care	3	3	5
Use of clinical registries	3	3	5

Abbreviations: BH, Behavioral health; BHI, Behavioral health integration; CPAP, Child Psychiatry Access Program; PCBH, Primary Care Behavioral Health; CoCM, Collaborative Care Model
Scale: 1-Not at all, 2-Rarely, 3-Sometimes, 4-Often, 5-Yes consistently.
[a] Based on screening or registry review.

plans are discussed in the context of consultation; however, CPAP teams, with some exceptions, rarely provide psychotherapy directly for patients within the pediatric practices.

Flexibility

The PCBH model may be considered the most flexible of the 3 models. The embedded behavioral health clinician can support population health by maintaining a systematic screening initiative, responding to immediate psychosocial crises, addressing health risk behaviors and behavioral health aspects of acute and chronic illness (with or without a formal psychiatric diagnosis), as well as providing brief psychotherapy, care coordination, and referrals. Any of these activities may or may not be included depending on practice interests and staffing availability. This flexibility allows practices to implement the PCBH model more easily than more highly-structured models such as the CoCM.

Funding

CPAPs are most commonly organized according to a geographic region (such as a state) and are sponsored by state and/or federal agencies. This makes the service "free" to individual primary care practices and allows the program to serve patients regardless of their insurance or ability to pay. In contrast, PCBH and CoCM program costs are usually directly borne by the primary care practice or network, and some or all of the costs are covered by some form of insurance reimbursement. As noted earlier, there are dedicated CPT codes that can be used to report charges associated with CoCM; however, utilization of these codes remains a barrier. Practice revenue from fee-for-service payments usually falls short of covering the total operational costs for PCBH and CoCM, and consequently, practices subsidize the gap, ideally through value-based payment mechanisms associated with commercial and/or public payors.

Population Health Focus

All 3 models are meant to support needs of a population of patients and therefore may be considered population health interventions. However, the population designed to be served by a CPAP ordinarily includes all children within a defined geographic region; whereas, the population served by a PCBH or CoCM program is a practice panel. All programs may carry out population health interventions such as supporting universal screening, working with patient registries, and other primary, secondary, and/or tertiary prevention initiatives; however, these functions are more consistently provided within CoCM implementations.

Education of the Primary Care Team

While all 3 models provide some degree of education regarding behavioral health to the primary care team, the CPAP model is the most explicitly educational in nature by virtue of its emphasis on telephonic interprofessional consultation. Lacking a direct relationship with the patient subject to the consultation and not having direct knowledge about the patient's history and presentation, the consultant's input is ordinarily framed as educational communication and information about best practices. Similarly, the consultant needs to emphasize that they are not directing any clinical decisions and that these decisions are entirely the responsibility of the PCP.

Involvement of a Child and Adolescent Psychiatrist

Both CPAPs and CoCM programs include a formal role for a child and adolescent psychiatrist, while having a child and adolescent psychiatrist available for consultation is an optional component of PCBH programs and is often not included. The role of the child and adolescent psychiatrist in participating in weekly review sessions with the BHCM is a novel and integral part of the CoCM. Similarly, the continuous availability of a child and adolescent psychiatrist for telephonic interprofessional consultation in CPAPs is a distinct feature and emphasis within this model.

Evidence Base/Clinical Effectiveness

All 3 models have been studied to some extent; however, the CoCM in general has been more rigorously studied with over 90 randomized controlled trials to date. As a result of this work, CoCM in general may be considered to have a stronger evidence base for clinical effectiveness. Given that there are significant differences between children and adults regarding clinical needs and practice settings, there needs to be continued work to adapt CoCM for pediatric settings and further clinical trials of implementation projects incorporating these adaptations need to be conducted. Given widespread adoption across the US there is increasing evidence supporting the CPAP model; however, most of the evidence to date has been focused on reception by primary care providers, feasibility, and engagement.[12]

SUMMARY

Integrating behavioral health services in pediatric primary care can help address the growing mental health needs of children and adolescents in the US. Given the different approaches for integration, pediatric primary care practices may evaluate the features of each model and considering tailoring it to their unique practice environments.

CLINICS CARE POINTS

- Three common models of integrating behavioral health services in pediatric primary care include: the Child Psychiatry Access Program model, the Primary Care Behavioral Health model, and the Collaborative Care Model.
- The Collaborative Care Model has a stronger evidence base for clinical effectiveness.
- There is increasing evidence supporting the Child Psychiatry Access Program model, though most of the evidence to date has been focused on user satisfaction, feasibility, and engagement.

DISCLOSURE

The authors have nothing to disclose.

FUNDING

Dr Lee and Dr Congdon were supported by funding from the National Center for Advancing Translational Sciences through UCSF-CTSI Grant Number KL2 TR001870.

REFERENCES

1. Bitsko RH, Claussen AH, Lichstein J, et al. Mental health surveillance among children—United States, 2013–2019. MMWR supplements 2022;71:1–42.
2. Racine N, McArthur BA, Cooke JE, et al. Global Prevalence of Depressive and Anxiety Symptoms in Children and Adolescents During COVID-19: A Meta-analysis. JAMA Pediatr 2021;175(11):1142–50.
3. AAP-AACAP-CHA Declaration of a National Emergency in Child and Adolescent Mental Health. American Academy of Pediatrics. 2021. Available at: https://www.aap.org/en/advocacy/child-and-adolescent-healthy-mental-development/aap-aacap-cha-declaration-of-a-national-emergency-in-child-and-adolescent-mental-health/. [Accessed 27 April 2024].
4. Office of the Surgeon G. Publications and Reports of the Surgeon General. Protecting youth mental health: the US Surgeon General's advisory. Washington, DC: US Department of Health and Human Services; 2021.
5. McBain RK, Kofner A, Stein BD, et al. Growth and Distribution of Child Psychiatrists in the United States: 2007-2016. Pediatrics 2019;144(6). https://doi.org/10.1542/peds.2019-1576.

6. Steinman KJ, Shoben AB, Dembe AE, et al. How long do adolescents wait for psychiatry appointments? Community Ment Health J 2015;51:782–9.
7. Hoffmann JA, Attridge MM, Carroll MS, et al. Association of Youth Suicides and County-Level Mental Health Professional Shortage Areas in the US. JAMA Pediatr 2023;177(1):71–80.
8. Bitsko RH, Holbrook JR, Robinson LR, et al. Health care, family, and community factors associated with mental, behavioral, and developmental disorders in early childhood—United States, 2011–2012. MMWR Morbidity and mortality weekly report 2016;65:221–6.
9. Green CM, Foy JM, Earls MF, et al. Achieving the pediatric mental health competencies. Pediatrics 2019;144(5). e20192758.
10. AACAP. Back to Project Future: Plan for the Coming Decade. Available at: https://www.aacap.org/App_Themes/AACAP/docs/member_resources/back_to_project_future/BPF_Plan_for_the_Coming_Decade_2014.pdf. [Accessed 5 May 2024].
11. Yonek J, Lee CM, Harrison A, et al. Key Components of Effective Pediatric Integrated Mental Health Care Models: A Systematic Review. JAMA Pediatr 2020;174(5):487–98.
12. Lee CM, Yonek J, Lin B, et al. Systematic Review: Child Psychiatry Access Program Outcomes. JAACAP Open 2023;1(3):154–72.
13. Sarvet B, Gold J, Bostic JQ, et al. Improving access to mental health care for children: the Massachusetts Child Psychiatry Access Project. Pediatrics 2010;126(6):1191–200.
14. NNCPAP. Child Psychiatry Access Programs in the United States. Available at: https://www.nncpap.org/map. [Accessed 25 March 2024].
15. HRSA. Pediatric Mental Health Care Access. Available at: https://mchb.hrsa.gov/programs-impact/programs/pediatric-mental-health-care-access. [Accessed 25 March 2024].
16. Sullivan K, George P, Horowitz K. Addressing National Workforce Shortages by Funding Child Psychiatry Access Programs. Pediatrics 2021;147(1). https://doi.org/10.1542/peds.2019-4012.
17. Gillies D, Buykx P, Parker AG, et al. Consultation liaison in primary care for people with mental disorders. Cochrane Database Syst Rev 2015;2015(9):CD007193.
18. Bettencourt AF, Plesko CM. A Systematic Review of the Methods Used to Evaluate Child Psychiatry Access Programs. Acad Pediatr 2020;20(8):1071–82.
19. Spencer AE, Platt RE, Bettencourt AF, et al. Implementation of Off-Site Integrated Care for Children: A Scoping Review. Harv Rev Psychiatry 2019;27(6):342–53.
20. Dvir Y, Straus JH, Sarvet B, et al. Key attributes of child psychiatry access programs. Perspective. Frontiers in Child and Adolescent Psychiatry 2023;2. https://doi.org/10.3389/frcha.2023.1244671.
21. Lee CM, Jeung J, Yonek JC, et al. Using human-centered design to develop and implement a pediatric mental health care access program. Community Case Study. Front Psychiatr 2024;14. https://doi.org/10.3389/fpsyt.2023.1283346.
22. Reiter JT, Dobmeyer AC, Hunter CL. The Primary Care Behavioral Health (PCBH) Model: An Overview and Operational Definition. J Clin Psychol Med Settings 2018;25(2):109–26.
23. Bodenheimer T, Sinsky C. From triple to quadruple aim: care of the patient requires care of the provider. Ann Fam Med 2014;12(6):573–6.
24. Cole MB, Qin Q, Sheldrick RC, et al. The effects of integrating behavioral health into primary care for low-income children. Health Serv Res 2019;54(6):1203–13.

25. Hostutler C, Wolf N, Snider T, et al. Increasing access to and utilization of behavioral health care through integrated primary care. Pediatrics 2023;152(6). e2023062514.
26. Hunter CL, Funderburk JS, Polaha J, et al. Primary Care Behavioral Health (PCBH) model research: Current state of the science and a call to action. J Clin Psychol Med Settings 2018;25:127–56.
27. Ngo VK, Asarnow JR, Lange J, et al. Outcomes for youths from racial-ethnic minority groups in a quality improvement intervention for depression treatment. Psychiatr Serv 2009;60(10):1357–64.
28. Weersing VR, Brent DA, Rozenman MS, et al. Brief behavioral therapy for pediatric anxiety and depression in primary care: a randomized clinical trial. JAMA Psychiatr 2017;74(6):571–8.
29. Asarnow JR, Rozenman M, Wiblin J, et al. Integrated Medical-Behavioral Care Compared With Usual Primary Care for Child and Adolescent Behavioral Health: A Meta-analysis. JAMA Pediatr 2015;169(10):929–37.
30. Walter HJ, Vernacchio L, Trudell EK, et al. Five-Year Outcomes of Behavioral Health Integration in Pediatric Primary Care. Pediatrics 2019;144(1). https://doi.org/10.1542/peds.2018-3243.
31. Foy JM, Green CM, Earls MF, Committee On Psychosocial Aspects Of C, Family Health MHLWG. Mental Health Competencies for Pediatric Practice. Pediatrics 2019;144(5). https://doi.org/10.1542/peds.2019-2757.
32. Horwitz SM, Storfer-Isser A, Kerker BD, et al. Barriers to the Identification and Management of Psychosocial Problems: Changes From 2004 to 2013. Acad Pediatr 2015;15(6):613–20.
33. Serrano N, Cordes C, Cubic B, et al. The state and future of the primary care behavioral health model of service delivery workforce. J Clin Psychol Med Settings 2018;25:157–68.
34. Tyler ET, Hulkower RL, Kaminski JW. Behavioral health integration in pediatric primary care. Milbank Memorial Fund 2017;15:1–24.
35. Lanoye A, Stewart KE, Rybarczyk BD, et al. The impact of integrated psychological services in a safety net primary care clinic on medical utilization. J Clin Psychol 2017;73(6):681–92.
36. Gouge N, Polaha J, Rogers R, et al. Integrating Behavioral Health into Pediatric Primary Care: Implications for Provider Time and Cost. South Med J 2016; 109(12):774–8.
37. Huffman JC, Niazi SK, Rundell JR, et al. Essential articles on collaborative care models for the treatment of psychiatric disorders in medical settings: a publication by the academy of psychosomatic medicine research and evidence-based practice committee. Psychosomatics 2014;55(2):109–22.
38. Reist C, Petiwala I, Latimer J, et al. Collaborative mental health care: a narrative review. Medicine 2022;101(52):e32554.
39. Ratzliff A, Unützer J, Katon W, et al. Integrated care: creating effective mental and primary health care teams. Hoboken, NJ: John Wiley & Sons; 2016.
40. Kroenke K, Unutzer J. Closing the false divide: sustainable approaches to integrating mental health services into primary care. J Gen Intern Med 2017;32(4): 404–10.
41. Heath B, Wise Romero, P., & Reynolds, K. A Standard Framework for Levels of Integrated Healthcare. 2013.

Integrated Behavioral Health

A Guide to Practical Implementation

Jessica M. McClure, PsyD[a,b,*], Melissa A. Young, PsyD[b,c]

KEYWORDS

• Integrated behavioral health • Primary care • Implementation

KEY POINTS

- Integrated behavioral health reduces barriers to care and is an accessible model for primary care practices.
- Resources and experts can be leveraged to support practices in implementing integrated behavioral health.
- Integrated behavioral health approaches vary in scope and models and can be customized to meet the needs of practices.

INTRODUCTION

The pediatric mental and behavioral health (MBH) crisis is undeniable, while the availability of effective evidence-based treatments (EBTs) is insufficient at best.[1,2] MBH needs of youth are soaring while access to care simultaneously declines, resulting in issues of inequity as many youth are unable to access the *right level of care* at the *right time*.[3–9] This leaves pediatric clinicians in primary care settings frequently serving as the main port of entry for youth experiencing MBH concerns.[10] With the majority of youth visiting a primary care provider yearly, and approximately 25% of these visits focused on addressing MBH concerns,[11–13] the pediatric primary care setting is well-suited for integrating MBH and physical health care.[14,15]

Under traditional referral systems, youth requiring specialty care (ie, MBH care outside of the primary care medical home via traditional outpatient services) often face additional barriers such as transportation, access, availability of appropriately trained MBH providers in the region, and lack of trust in an external system.[16] When

[a] Population Behavioral Health, Office of Population Health; [b] Division of Behavioral Medicine and Clinical Psychology, Cincinnati Children's Hospital Medical Center, 3333 Burnet Avenue, MLC 15018, Cincinnati, OH 45229, USA; [c] Department of Pediatrics, University of Cincinnati College of Medicine, Cincinnati, OH, USA
* Corresponding author. 3333 Burnet Avenue, MLC 15018, Cincinnati, OH 45229.
E-mail address: jessica.mcclure@cchmc.org

Pediatr Clin N Am 71 (2024) 1073–1086
https://doi.org/10.1016/j.pcl.2024.07.014 pediatric.theclinics.com
0031-3955/24/

MBH and physical health needs are addressed within the primary care setting, families report feeling more comfortable with initiating treatment, the treatment team is more informed about how MBH treatment is progressing, and treatment can be accessed more efficiently and effectively within the medical home.[17]

Despite the opportunity to integrate physical and MBH in the medical home, pediatric clinicians within primary care settings often report uncertainty around identification and treatment initiation for MBH concerns.[18,19] While programs have evolved to provide more comprehensive training for pediatric clinicians, fully treating MBH symptoms in isolation is less than ideal.

Integrated behavioral health (IBH) within the primary care setting has been shown to reduce barriers to care, thereby reducing the adverse impact of disparities surrounding access.[15,20] However, solely embedding an MBH provider within a primary care clinic is not enough, as there are key components essential to the development, implementation, and sustainability of an effective IBH program. Within large hospital systems, this is typically obtained through leveraging the expertise of subject matter experts with MBH leaders overseeing integrated programs. However, for smaller systems or individual practices, the challenges of setting up an IBH model may be greater. Thus, the purpose of this study is to guide pediatric clinicians seeking to develop and implement an IBH program in their clinics. Specifically, the elements of a comprehensive IBH program will be outlined and commonly asked questions addressed.

Elements of a Comprehensive Integrated Behavioral Health Program

Embedding MBH services within an individual primary care practice can be overwhelming. MBH scheduling, billing, vetting candidates, and identifying appropriate MBH clinical outcome measurements are often new to pediatric clinicians.[18] Pediatric clinicians and practices are encouraged to use existing resources and expertise in their region to fill the gaps in knowledge or capacity of their practice. Leveraging regional expertise not only reduces the burden on the individual practice but also can foster the development of a network of practices that share resources, which affords the MBH providers a cohort of colleagues for collaboration and consultation while reducing provider burnout and improving retention.[21]

Pediatric clinicians often ask, where do I start?

An IBH program can be implemented in a variety of ways and provide a range of MBH services. The first step when considering IBH for your practice is to determine the existing capacity and level of expertise in the practice, as well as options for filling any existing gaps in those areas (**Box 1**). Feasibility will inevitably vary based on the clinic's existing infrastructure and resources that can be leveraged to support the initial design, development, and implementation of IBH for that practice. An IBH program can start by launching one service line and expand to additional services over time. The range of services should be tailored to the setting and needs of the practice, billing options in the clinic's state, and availability of resources.

Should my practice go it alone or partner with an academic medical center or other organization?

Questions regarding your practice's capacity and capability are outlined in **Box 1** followed by suggested partnership tiers with IBH program design and implementation experts, which will help determine the best way to proceed.

What model of integration would meet the needs of our practice?

Leaders must decide which form of integration will initially be the most feasible and sustainable for their practice. There are 3 types of integration according to the

Box 1
Practice capacity

What scope of work does my practice have the expertise and/or capacity to initially manage?

- Do we have identified criteria for an IBH role (eg, types of presenting concerns and services that will be within the scope of the selected IBH model)?
- Do we offer a salary range and benefits that will attract candidates?
- Does our practice include someone with extensive knowledge of evidence-based MBH treatments to thoroughly evaluate prospective candidates' understanding and use of EBTs?
- Does our practice include someone with knowledge of expected outcomes for EBTs and MBC approaches for pediatric IBH to sufficiently oversee the clinical model and outcomes?
- Do we have someone in our practice who understands credentialing, billing, and scheduling standards for MBH?

If you answered no to any of these questions, your practice may want to consider partnering with experts in IBH program design and implementation. Examples of partnerships may include

- A one-time consultation with a subject matter expert to gather information necessary to expand the practice's internal capacity and expertise.
- Development of a consultative relationship with leaders of an existing IBH program to assist with leveraging internal expertise for program development and implementation.
- Engagement in full partnership with an expert team to lead the development and implementation of IBH with input from the practice.

Substance Abuse and Mental Health Services Administration Center for Integrated Health Solutions, which include coordinated care, colocated care, and integrated care.[22] Coordinated care is consistent with typical outpatient services where MBH providers and pediatric clinicians practice in separate systems and occasionally communicate about their patients. In contrast, colocated refers to MBH providers and pediatric clinicians practicing within the same facility. Colocated services are further delineated based on whether systems and processes are shared among MBH providers and pediatric clinicians. Integrated care allows patients to receive seamless care from MBH providers and pediatric clinicians within a shared space.[22] In addition to identifying the level of integration, practice leaders must consider this decision within the context of financial resources and models within their state (eg, reimbursement rates for billed services vary by IBH provider type, insurance payor, and state). While colocated services can be easier to sustain financially in the short term, fully integrated services afford long-term benefits to patients while demonstrating an increased financial sustainability over time.[23,24] Further, patient volumes and the full-time equivalent (FTE) of the IBH provider are additional factors that must be considered. To illustrate, a practice predominantly delivering care to adolescents and young adults (AYAs) may initially focus on colocated services (ie, including crisis stabilization due to the ongoing youth MBH crisis) before implementing integrated, preventative services.

Which integrated behavioral health services should we initially launch?

Identifying the needs of your patient population and the capacity of your practice is essential to determine which services to initially offer. For example, practices with a lar nfant and early childhood patient population may choose to focus on developing prevention service line before expanding offerings for intervention and crisis on, as these typically are geared toward school-aged children and adoles- types of service are commonly offered as part of a comprehensive IBH se services include[1] prevention,[2] intervention,[3] crisis assessment and am and resident education, and[5] outcome measurement and program evaluation[25–27] and are outlined in **Table 1**. Care coordination is also an important component of an IBH program. Care coordination services can be delivered by another team member and/or by the MBH provider and can assist families in identifying and connecting with appropriate resources and services.[19]

Prevention. Prevention services can be implemented across the pediatric lifespan; however, these services are often geared toward children aged from birth through 5 years.[28–32] While prevention services typically target infants and young children, it is important to consider providing these services to AYAs. Prevention services can be offered universally at the practice population level (eg, every youth within the designated age range is eligible for IBH prevention services) or can be offered to families following a screening that identifies specific risks or needs.

Intervention. Variability in the quality and effectiveness of MBH services can lead to poor patient outcomes and higher rates of emergency department (ED) utilization or inpatient psychiatric admissions when symptoms escalate or a crisis occurs.[6,33–35] Therefore, the delivery of effective evidence-based MBH intervention is essential, as this improves patient outcomes, which leads to shorter lengths of treatment and availability for new patients to access care via the IBH program.[1,36] Cognitive behavioral therapy (CBT) is regarded as the gold standard evidence-based psychotherapy for a host of MBH concerns.[37] CBT is based on the premise that changes to thoughts, behaviors, and/or body sensations result in changes to emotional functioning.[38] While CBT is typically the first choice, other psychotherapies are considered evidence-based for specific presenting concerns. For example, both CBT and interpersonal psychotherapy are regarded as appropriate EBTs for adolescent depression. These intervention models can be applied via IBH, increasing patient and family access to effective care while also increasing collaboration and coordination of care between the IBH and pediatric clinician.

Crisis stabilization. In the context of the ongoing youth MBH crisis, it is important to consider including crisis stabilization services as part of the IBH model. Comprehensive crisis stabilization services ideally extend beyond the IBH provider to incorporate processes that the practice's staff can follow when safety concerns arise to ensure that youth receive the care needed while also not unnecessarily being referred to the ED.[6] The *Blueprint for Youth Suicide Prevention* is an excellent resource that includes recommendations and a clinical pathway based on the best available research evidence for universal suicide screening (Ask Suicide-Screening Questions), assessment (Brief Suicide Safety Assessment), and intervention within the pediatric primary care setting.[39] Additionally, the *Stanley Brown Safety Plan* is a well-researched safety planning tool that can be easily utilized by pediatric clinicians and/or IBH providers when concerns surrounding suicidality arise.[40]

Team and resident education. IBH providers are uniquely poised to provide continuing education opportunities (eg, didactics, case presentations, modeling/role-playing interventions, and so forth) for team members, which can occur during existing meetings or the lunch hour. Initially, educational content should focus on aspects of clinical care that pediatric clinicians may be less comfortable addressing (eg, safety planning, obsessive-compulsive disorder, and so forth) yet are commonly seen within the practice. IBH providers can offer curbside consults or structured case consultations (eg, biweekly case consultation groups) to clinician colleagues and resident pediatric clinicians to increase knowledge and self-efficacy surrounding the management of pediatric MBH concerns. IBH providers can also serve an integral role

Table 1
Services across the continuum of integrated behavioral health care

Service	Description	Advantages	Challenges
Prevention	Integration of MBH services into well visits. Prevention-focused MBH services expand upon Bright Future Guidelines	Universal prevention programs have been found to reduce future MBH concerns while building trust and connection to the medical home	Clinicians may initially prioritize the care of youth with higher acuity MBH concerns Reimbursement for preventive services varies across states and payors
Intervention	Targeted, EBT for MBH concerns	Quick access to effective evidence-based care that reduces treatment duration and the need for higher levels of care	Some families, clinicians, and MBH providers are less familiar with the episodic delivery of EBTs and therefore seek longer term supportive counseling
Crisis assessment and stabilization	Provision of evidence-based screening, assessment, and intervention for crises/safety concerns offered within the medical home	Reduces utilization of higher levels of care while offering expedited access to evidence-based care to address safety concerns Provides care in a convenient and trusted environment while reducing stress and health care costs for the family	Processes are needed to identify safety concerns and to quickly connect patients to the IBH provider, including processes for crisis management when IBH provider is unavailable
Team and resident education	Training for clinicians and other team members on EBTs for common pediatric MBH concerns, motivational interviewing, safety assessments, and so forth	The IBH provider will be aware of practice culture and processes, so they can develop brief-focused training tailored to the needs of clinicians and staff in the practice Training can be integrated into existing meetings or offered during the lunch hour	Time and resources will need to be allocated to ensure the IBH provider has sufficient time to develop training opportunities that are meaningful for clinicians and other relevant personnel
Program and clinical outcome evaluation	Standardized method for evaluating outcomes at the patient and program level	Allows practice leaders, clinicians, and IBH providers to evaluate outcomes, which can be shared with patients, families, and other stakeholders	Depending on the practice's existing resources, additional financial, personnel, and operational support may be needed to obtain reliable data to measure outcomes

resident training. Resident physicians can shadow IBH providers to diversify their experiences during medical rotations. IBH providers can also precept with resident physicians on MBH aspects of a patient's care.[41,42]

Outcome measurement and program evaluation. Several measures can be used to evaluate various aspects of an IBH program, including clinical outcomes, satisfaction, and financial sustainability. To examine patient-level and population-level clinical outcomes, it is important to identify a measure that can be used with a wide range of presenting problems/diagnoses and be easily administered at every IBH session, which is consistent with a measurement-based care (MBC) approach to MBH treatment.[25] At the programmatic level, the focus of evaluation measure will vary based on the element that is being evaluated. For example, the rate of patients who present to the ED for MBH concerns can be used as a proxy for evaluating the effectiveness of the crisis stabilization service, whereas the number of new visits (ie, representing new, unique patients entering MBH treatment) per month could be used for evaluating access to the IBH service. Other outcome measures can be utilized to align with broader practice priorities (eg, HEDIS metrics, clinician satisfaction, and patient/family experience). Revenue generated by billing for IBH services can be evaluated in comparison to the overall cost of the IBH program to measure the financial sustainability of the program. **Table 2** outlines potential outcome measures and how the information can inform program evaluation.

Do we need a full-time or part-time integrated behavioral health provider?

While pediatric clinician and/or practice panel size is often used to determine the initial FTE needed for IBH, solely focusing on panel size fails to account for other factors that can significantly impact IBH patient volumes and, therefore, financial sustainability. These factors include seasonal fluctuations, the rate of pediatric clinicians referring patients to the IBH service, and the type of IBH services offered (eg, prevention, crisis stabilization, and so forth).

Tracking referral volume for a few weeks as part of the preplanning for IBH can help practice leaders identify *current* MBH needs of their practice; however, it is important to keep in mind that referral volumes tend to shift seasonally and longitudinally.[43,44] Regarding referral rates, when an IBH program is initially launched, many pediatric clinicians will quickly identify and refer youth with moderate-to-severe MBH concerns while they may initially be less likely to refer youth with mild or subclinical concerns. Thus, initial referral estimates will typically underestimate patient volumes that may be seen after the IBH program has been launched for some time (**Table 3**). Efforts focused on educating pediatric clinicians and other team members on the type and scope of IBH services should be prioritized at the launch of the program and occasionally thereafter (eg, quarterly), based on patient volumes and the capacity of the IBH provider.

In addition to these referral volume considerations, a comprehensive understanding of practice needs is essential. Conducting a thorough readiness assessment at the practice level while planning to launch an IBH program can be used to develop projections of initial referral volume and patterns, which can provide additional data when deciding whether a full-time or part-time FTE is needed. The readiness assessment can be completed by the practice champion (ie, the clinician who is actively engaged in the development and implementation of the IBH program) to help direct this decision. Various versions of practice readiness assessments exist (eg, Readiness for Integrated Care Questionnaire[45]), and a sample version has been included here as well (**Fig. 1**).

Table 2
Practice-level outcome measures

Measures	Description	Purpose
MBH ED and inpatient admissions	Rate of ED visits and inpatient admissions for MBH per 1000 patients at the practice	Measure the effectiveness of IBH crisis stabilization services at the practice level
HEDIS	Percentage of patients who were seen for follow-up within 7 and 30 d following an MBH ED visit or inpatient admission	Ensure meaningful follow-up occurs within specified time frames after a mental health crisis (eg, ED or inpatient admission)
Financial sustainability	Revenue generated by IBH billed services in comparison to IBH operating costs	Identify opportunities to modify IBH model to maximize sustainability based on revenue trends
Access	Number of new IBH patient visits scheduled per month	Monitor patient access to the IBH service, ensure the IBH program is appropriately sized for the practice, and identify unmet needs or opportunities for expansion
Patient and family satisfaction	Routine collection of patient and family experiences	Measure the impact of the IBH program on changes to patient and family satisfaction, which can then be shared with clinicians and other key interested parties[37]
Clinician satisfaction	Routine collection of pediatric clinician satisfaction and/or burnout	Measure impact of IBH program on pediatric clinician satisfaction pre-embedding/postembedding IBH services and routinely thereafter[38,39]
Symptom-specific screeners (eg, PHQ-A, GAD-7, and so forth)	Patient-level symptom screeners commonly used in pediatric primary care	Monitor positive screening rates at the population level to inform treatment planning[40]

Abbreviations: ED, emergency department; GAD-7, Generalized Anxiety Disorder-7th Edition; HEDIS, Health Plan Employer Data and Information Set; MBH, mental and behavioral health; PHQ-A, Patient Health Questionnaire Modified for Teens.

Table 3
Common referral patterns

Referral Patterns <0–6 mo	Referral Patterns >6–12 mo
• Moderate to severe concerns for depression, anxiety, and ADHD • Disruptive behavior and tantrums • School avoidance, refusal, and/or truancy • Suicidality and/or nonsuicidal self-injury	• Emerging or mild MBH concerns • Self-regulation symptoms for young children (eg, sleep difficulties, potty training, needle fear, picky eating, and so forth) • Emerging externalizing concerns (eg, aggression) • Trauma

What are the common referral patterns during the first year of the IBH program?

Two practices of equivalent size may have different referral volumes and patterns depending on factors such as location, availability of community MBH resources, pediatric clinicians' knowledge/comfort in treating MBH conditions, and the age range of patients seen in the practice. Further, practices that adopt universal MBH prevention

Behavioral Health Needs
Practice Readiness Assessment

Practice Name: ____________

Date Completed: ____________

Completed by: ____________

Demographic Information:

		Hours of operation	
# of Active Patients in Practice	______		
# of Physicians in Practice	______	______	Monday
# of APRNs in Practice	______	______	Tuesday
# of PAs in Practice	______	______	Wednesday
# of Practice Sites/Locations	______	______	Thursday
Average # of WCC per day	______	______	Friday
Average # of total visits per day	______	______	Saturday
No show rate	______	______	Sunday
Electronic Medical Record in Use	______		
Commercial Insurance Payor %	______	Medicaid Payor %	______

Primary Practice Contact Name: ______ Email: ______ Phone: ______

Physician Champion Name: ______ Email: ______ Phone: ______

What current screening tools are being used in the Practice?

#1	____________	Age(s) administered	______
#2	____________	Age(s) administered	______
#3	____________	Age(s) administered	______
#4	____________	Age(s) administered	______
#5	____________	Age(s) administered	______
#6	____________	Age(s) administered	______

Clinical Needs/Services

1 - Please describe the behavioral health needs of the patients and families in your practice.

2 - What behavioral health resources/services do you currently offer within the practice?

3 - What behavioral health resources/referrals do you recommend for patients/families (off

Fig. 1. Sample Practice Readiness Form.

site/outside of practice)?

4 - Please describe your vision for how a behavioral health specialist would integrate into your practice, treat patients and families, and collaborate and coordinate care with the medical team.

5- In the chart below please indicate the # of patients per week that are seen in your practice and would benefit from a behavioral health consultation or follow up visit by a behavioral health specialist:

Presenting Concern	0-2 Years Old	2-5 Years Old	6-12 Years Old	13-18 Years Old	Young Adults	Caregivers of Patients
Anxiety/phobias/OCD						
Depression						
Suicidality						
Self-injury						
ADHD evaluation						
ADHD treatment						
Behavioral concerns						
School Problems						
Adjustment Issues						
Feeding/weight management						
Sleep concerns						
Pill swallowing						
Pain/Headaches						
Other:						
Other:						

Operational Considerations

1 - We have the patient volume to support a full time behavioral health provider: Yes/No

2 – We have the financial flexibility to ramp up a new behavioral health provider over a 3–4-month time: Yes/No

3 - What space is available for the behavioral health specialist to use when seeing patients?

4 - What space is available for the behavioral health specialist to use for charting/office work?

5 - Please describe your current telehealth services and how you envision behavioral health utilizing telehealth options?

6- We have a staff member with dedicated time to facilitate the set up and onboarding of the behavioral health specialist (e.g., credentialing, updating electronic health record/note templates, scheduling behavioral health patients, developing written materials for patients/families about cost/services)

Specific staff member(s) dedicated to onboarding and amount of time per week allocated:

Fig. 1. (*continued*).

and early intervention may initially be able to sustain a higher level of FTE than a larger practice that only utilizes IBH for moderate-to-severe mental health concerns, which illustrates the importance of considering the results of the needs assessment within the context of designing the IBH program.

How can I ensure the integrated behavioral health program is financially sustainable? Financial sustainability of IBH is dynamic and depends on the nuances of the region, practice, and the type of IBH model within the practice.[46] At the outset of program implementation, practice leaders should ensure that there are approximately 3 to 6 months of financial resources available to cover personnel and programmatic costs, as the IBH provider will not generate sufficient revenue to cover these expenses at the outset. Other considerations surrounding financial sustainability include reimbursement rates, average no-show rate for the practice, and patient volume needed to cover personnel and operational costs. See **Box 2**, for additional considerations.

Throughout the lifespan of the IBH program, there may be times when patient volumes are low (eg, in the case of expected seasonality trends). Over time, these trends will become apparent and practice leaders can proactively expand the scope of IBH during expected periods when patient volumes are low (**Box 3** for additional ideas). Outside of maximizing the reach of IBH, financial sustainability can also be addressed in some systems through grants, philanthropic funds, or partnerships with larger health systems that will reduce the financial burden on individual practices. For example, multiple practices may consider partnering on and sharing IBH providers or collaborating with an outside behavioral health organization to provide IBH services.

DISCUSSION

While there are numerous benefits for patients, families, and pediatric clinicians, there are many factors to consider before launching an IBH program. Practice leaders and

Box 2
Initial and longitudinal financial stability

These questions can be used by practice leaders and clinicians to determine key elements that may impact the initial and longitudinal financial sustainability of an IBH program.

- Are there limitations on which mental health-related codes can be billed (ie, different reimbursement rates) by the IBH provider type we are aiming to hire?
- What is the average reimbursement rate for the mental health-related codes we plan to include in our IBH model? If the payor mix is diverse, this will need to be factored into the calculations.
- At the identified rates, how many visits would an IBH provider need to bill (ie, per day, week, month, and year) for the program to be financially sustainable? Is that a realistic number? Does that account for time out of the office for vacation/sick days and time for nonbillable services?
- What is the practice's average no-show rate? How will no-shows impact financial sustainability?
- What patient volume (eg, 5 billable hours a day) would be needed to cover 100% of salary, benefits, and overhead costs (if additional funding is not available to offset these costs)?
- What is the cost of salary, benefits, and overhead for a full-time versus part-time provider? Can we support the salary, benefits, and overhead costs for a full-time provider for 3 to 6 months following program launch? If not, can we support a part-time provider?
- Who will serve as the clinician champion for the IBH program? Will the clinician champion require dedicated time to support the launch and ongoing implementation of the IBH program? If yes, what dedicated FTE will the clinician champion need?

Box 3
Referrals and patient volumes

How can practices maximize the scope of referrals after launching the IBH program?

- Identify a referral focus for the day or week to raise clinician awareness of that type of presenting concern. For example, clinicians focus on identifying and referring patients with concerns of mild/subclinical depression, sleep disturbance, or mealtime behavior concerns to the IBH provider.
- The IBH provider hosts monthly lunch and learn sessions on a specific topic, which could include case examples and quotes/comments from pediatric clinicians who are early adopters of the IBH program.
- The practice develops a quality improvement initiative focused on improving patient outcomes at the population level. For example, an intervention could take the form of connecting patients to the IBH provider within 30 days following a positive depression screen during annual well visits.
- Practices obtain routine feedback from patients and families to share with the team during monthly staff meetings.
- The IBH provider shadows pediatric clinicians and provides real-time feedback on additional supports and services they could provide based on the clinical encounter.

pediatric clinicians are encouraged to consult or partner with experts before launching a program. Consulting or partnering with regional experts in IBH program development and implementation allows independent practices to leverage learnings from other programs, including regarding what models of care have been successful in that region/state. While this study provides practical guidance for implementation of IBH in community primary care settings, it is important to recognize that regional or local variations in workforce availability, reimbursement rates, and other levels of MBH care available in the surrounding community will be important considerations.

SUMMARY

The need for and benefits of increased integration of MBH and physical health care for youth is clear, yet the logistics of initiating an IBH program at the practice level can be overwhelming and pose barriers to smaller, independent practices. By employing established guidelines, local resources, and subject matter experts and taking a gradual and planful approach, pediatric clinicians can set their practices up to succeed in this model of care. Key decision points for practices include whether or not to partner with an outside organization to standup an IBH model, what model of integration and what levels of MBH care to offer through IBH, whether a full-time or part-time IBH provider will meet the practice's needs, and whether the IBH program can be financially sustainable.

CLINICS CARE POINTS

- Pediatric primary care IBH programs increase timely access to MBH care for patients and families within the medical home.
- Primary care leaders and pediatric clinicians are encouraged to consult with existing IBH program leaders and other experts in their region.
- Identifying the needs of the patient population and the capacity of the practice is essential for choosing which IBH services to launch and the model of integration.
- Outcome measurement at the patient, population, and practice level is important for monitoring clinical outcomes, provider and family satisfaction, and financial sustainability.

- IBH within the primary care setting has been shown to reduce many barriers to care, thereby reducing the adverse impact of disparities surrounding access.
- IBH increases families' comfort initiating MBH treatment, the pediatric clinicians are more informed about how MBH treatment is progressing, and MBH treatment can be accessed more efficiently and effectively within the medical home.

DISCLOSURE

The authors have nothing to disclose.

REFERENCES

1. Gyani A, Shafran R, Myles P, et al. The gap between science and practice: How therapists make their clinical decisions. Behav Ther 2014;45(2):199–211.
2. Meyer AE, Rodriguez-Quintana N, Miner K, et al. Developing a statewide network of coaches to support youth access to evidence-based practices. Implement Res Pract 2022;3:26334895221101215.
3. Abrams AH, Badolato GM, Boyle MD, et al. Racial and ethnic disparities in pediatric mental health-related emergency department visits. Pediatr Emerg Care 2022;38(1):e214–8.
4. Baams L. Disparities for LGBTQ and gender nonconforming adolescents. Pediatrics 2018;141(5). e20173004.
5. Brewer AG, Doss W, Sheehan KM, et al. Trends in suicidal ideation-related emergency department visits for youth in Illinois: 2016-2021. Pediatrics 2022;150(6). e2022056793.
6. Kalb LG, Stapp EK, Ballard ED, et al. Trends in psychiatric emergency department visits among youth and young adults in the US. Pediatrics 2019;143(4): e20182192.
7. Institute of Medicine (US) Committee on Quality of Health Care in America. Crossing the quality chasm: a new health system for the 21st century. Washington (DC): National Academies Press (US); 2001.
8. Hoffmann JA, Alegria M, Alvarez K, et al. Disparities in pediatric mental and behavioral health conditions. Pediatrics 2022;150(4). e2022058227.
9. Lau A, Barnett M, Stadnick N, et al. Therapist report of adaptations to delivery of evidence-based practices within a system-driven reform of publicly funded children's mental health services. J Consult Clin Psychol 2017;85(7):664–75.
10. Tobin-Tyler EH, Hulkower RL, Kaminski JW. Behavioral health integration in pediatric primary care: Considerations and opportunities for policymakers, planners, and providers. Available at: https://www.milbank.org/resources/, Milbank Memorial Fund, (Accessed December 16 2023). 2017.
11. Cooper S, Valleley RJ, Polaha J, et al. Running out of time: Physician management of behavioral health concerns in rural pediatric primary care. Pediatrics 2006;118(1):e132–8.
12. Kelleher KJ, Stevens J. Evolution of child mental health services in primary care. Acad Pediatr 2009;9(1):7–14.
13. Polaha J, Dalton WT, Allen S. The prevalence of emotional and behavior problems in pediatric primary care serving rural children. J Pediatr Psychol 2011;36(6): 652–60.
14. Brino KAS. Pediatric mental health and the power of primary care: Practical approaches and validating challenges. J Pediatr Health Care 2020;34(2):e12–20.

15. Asarnow JR, Rozenman M, Wiblin J, et al. Integrated medical-behavioral care compared with usual primary care for child and adolescent behavioral health: A meta-analysis. JAMA Pediatr 2015;169(10):929–37.
16. de Soet R, Vermeiren R, Bansema CH, et al. Drop-out and ineffective treatment in youth with severe and enduring mental health problems: A systematic review. Eur Child Adolesc Psychiatry 2023;1–15.
17. Schneider M, Mehari K, Langhinrichsen-Rohling J. What caregivers want: Preferences for behavioral health screening implementation procedures in pediatric primary care. J Clin Psychol Med Settings 2021;28(3):562–74.
18. Brady KJS, Durham MP, Francoeur A, et al. Barriers and facilitators to integrating behavioral health services and primary care. Clin Pract Pediatr Psychol 2021; 9(4):359–71.
19. McMillan JA, Land M Jr, Tucker AE, et al. Preparing future pediatricians to meet the behavioral and mental health needs of children. Pediatrics 2020;145(1): e20183796.
20. Parikh MR, O'Dell SM, Cook LA, et al. Integrated care is associated with increased behavioral health access and utilization for youth in crisis. Fam Syst Health 2021;39(3):426–33.
21. McClure JM, Merk FL, Anderson J, et al. Expanding access to cognitive behavioral therapy: A purposeful and effective model for integration. Cogn Behav Pract 2023;31(3):286–98.
22. Scharf DM, Eberhart NK, Hackbarth NS, et al. Evaluation of the SAMHSA primary and behavioral health care integration (PBHCI) grant program: Final report. Rand Health Q 2014;4(3):6.
23. Cummings AD, Van Horne B, Correa N, et al. Can pediatric primary care practices afford integrated behavioral health? A comparison of 5 pediatric practices. Clin Pediatr (Phila) 2022;61(12):850–8.
24. Herbst RB, Margolis KL, McClellan BB, et al. Sustaining integrated behavioral health practice without sacrificing the continuum of care. Clin Pract Pediatr Psychol 2018;6(2):117–28.
25. Barber J, Resnick SG. Collect, Share, Act: A transtheoretical clinical model for doing measurement-based care in mental health treatment. Psychol Serv 2023; 20(Suppl 2):150–7.
26. Boswell JF, Hepner KA, Lysell K, et al. The need for a measurement-based care professional practice guideline. Psychotherapy (Chic) 2023;60(1):1–16.
27. Jensen-Doss A, Douglas S, Phillips DA, et al. Measurement-based care as a practice improvement tool: Clinical and organizational applications in youth mental health. Evid Based Pract Child Adolesc Ment Health 2020;5(3):233–50.
28. Boyle CL, Sanders MR, Lutzker JR, et al. An analysis of training, generalization, and maintenance effects of Primary Care Triple P for parents of preschool-aged children with disruptive behavior. Child Psychiatr Hum Dev 2010;41(1):114–31.
29. Briggs RD, Silver EJ, Krug LM, et al. Healthy steps as a moderator: The impact of maternal trauma on child social-emotional development. Clin Pract Pediatr Psychol 2014;2(2):166–75.
30. Briggs RD, Stettler EM, Silver EJ, et al. Social-emotional screening for infants and toddlers in primary care. Pediatrics 2012;129(2):e377–84.
31. Ammerman RT, Rybak TM, Herbst RB, et al. Integrated behavioral health prevention for infants in pediatric primary care: A mixed-methods pilot study. J Pediatr Psychol 2024;49(4):298–308.

32. Raglin Bignall WJ, Herbst RB, McClure JM, et al. Adapting a preschool disruptive behavior group for the underserved in pediatric primary care practice. Fam Syst Health 2023;41(1):101–11.
33. Curtin SC. State suicide rates among adolescents and young adults aged 10-24: United States, 2000-2018. Natl Vital Stat Rep 2020;69(11):1–10.
34. Curtin SC, Garnett MF and Ahmad FB. Provisional numbers and rates of suicide by month and demographic characteristics: United States, 2020, Available at: www.cdc.gov/nchs/products/index.htm, (Accessed December 16 2023). 2021.
35. MacDonald K, Laporte L, Desrosiers L, et al. Emergency department use for mental health problems by youth in child welfare services. J Can Acad Child Adolesc Psychiatry 2022;31(4):202–13.
36. Herschell AD, Kolko DJ, Hart JA, et al. Mixed method study of workforce turnover and evidence-based treatment implementation in community behavioral health care settings. Child Abuse Negl 2020;102:104419.
37. David D, Cristea I, Hofmann SG. Why cognitive behavioral therapy is the current gold standard of psychotherapy. Front Psychiatry 2018;9:4.
38. Beck JS. Cognitive behavior therapy: basics and beyond. 3rd edition. New York: The Guilford Press; 2021.
39. Aguinaldo LD, Sullivant S, Lanzillo EC, et al. Validation of the ask suicide-screening questions (ASQ) with youth in outpatient specialty and primary care clinics. Gen Hosp Psychiatry 2021;68:52–8.
40. Stanley BB GK. Safety planning intervention: A brief intervention to mitigate suicide risk. Cogn Behav Pract 2012;19(2):256–64.
41. Pisani AR, leRoux P, Siegel DM. Educating residents in behavioral health care and collaboration: integrated clinical training of pediatric residents and psychology fellows. Acad Med 2011;86(2):166–73.
42. Tolliver M, Dueweke AR, Polaha J. Interprofessional microteaching: An innovation to strengthen the behavioral health competencies of the primary care workforce. Fam Syst Health 2022;40(4):484–90.
43. Walter HJ, Vernacchio L, Trudell EK, et al. Five-year outcomes of behavioral health integration in pediatric primary care. Pediatrics 2019;144(1):e20183243.
44. Vechiu C, Zimmermann M, Zepeda M, et al. Referral patterns and sociodemographic predictors of adult and pediatric behavioral health referrals in a Federally Qualified Health Center. J Behav Health Serv Res 2024;51(1):101–13.
45. Scott VC, Kenworthy T, Godly-Reynolds E, et al. The Readiness for Integrated Care Questionnaire (RICQ): An instrument to assess readiness to integrate behavioral health and primary care. Am J Orthopsychiatry 2017;87(5):520–30.
46. Muse AR, Lamson AL, Didericksen KW, et al. A systematic review of evaluation research in integrated behavioral health care: Operational and financial characteristics. Fam Syst Health 2017;35(2):136–54.

Pediatric Mental Health Prevention Programs in Primary Care

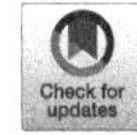

Yu Chen, PhD*, Danruo Zhong, PhD, Erin Roby, PhD, Caitlin Canfield, PhD, Alan Mendelsohn, MD

KEYWORDS

• Pediatrics • Mental health • Prevention program • Early childhood • Primary care

KEY POINTS

- Pediatric primary care has offered important venues to integrate mental and behavioral health services for children and their families.
- Six selected innovative approaches in prevention programs in pediatric care demonstrated recent research and clinical efforts in engaging families and promoting mental health in young children.
- For better prevention outcomes, future clinical practice should incorporate a broader engagement of family members, especially the father, and integrate strategies addressing perinatal maternal mental health, such that children's mental health risks can be mitigated before birth.

INTRODUCTION

One in six children aged 2 to 8 years is diagnosed with mental, behavioral, or developmental disorders.[1–3] Mental health problems in infancy and early childhood predict and contribute to adult mental health issues, leading to profound life-long consequences including occupational impairments, increased substance use, reduced quality of life, and adverse health outcomes (eg, chronic diseases and cancer).,[4–6]

The American Academy of Pediatrics (AAP)[7] has endorsed a paradigm shift toward early relational health (ERH), a framework that emphasizes the significance of safe, stable, and nurturing relationships that buffer childhood adversity and support healthy development and mental health.[6] Indeed, early positive child-caregiver relationships are associated with optimal cognitive development, social competence, and behavioral adjustment.[7,8] Translating this relational health framework into clinical practice, pediatric primary care has offered important venues to integrate mental and

Division of Developmental-Behavioral Pediatrics, Department of Pediatrics, NYU Grossman School of Medicine, 462 1st Avenue, OBV A529, New York, NY 10016, USA
* Corresponding author.
E-mail address: Yu.Chen2@nyulangone.org

Pediatr Clin N Am 71 (2024) 1087–1099
https://doi.org/10.1016/j.pcl.2024.07.015 pediatric.theclinics.com
0031-3955/24/

behavioral health services for children and their families given its accessibility, low cost, familiar providers, and nonstigmatizing environments.[9–11]

Nevertheless, recent years have presented new challenges that pose threats to children's mental health, such as widening disparities in health, education, and economics in the context of structural racism, and isolation caused by the coronavirus disease 2019 (COVID-19) pandemic,[12,13] which underscore the need for innovative approaches in primary care settings. This article presents 6 innovative approaches in prevention programs in pediatric care. Note that the selected approaches and programs serve as examples to illustrate innovative developments in this field. More comprehensive lists can be found elsewhere.[9,10,14]

Relationship-Based Approaches in Primary Care

Recently, relationship-based approaches, which focus on interventionist-mother/family relationships, and parent-child relationships during preventive sessions have been used by pediatric mental health preventive programs in primary care.[15] Unlike didactic approaches where practitioners act as educators, pinpointing caregivers' weaknesses in child-rearing, relationship-based approaches prioritize empathy. That is, interventionists partner with families, actively listening and honoring parents as experts on their children, and help identify, clarify, and address issues that may impact parents' developing relationships with their children.[15] Such strategies increase family coping skills, support positive family relationships, and build resilience in mental health in children and caregivers.[16,17]

PlayReadVIP

PlayReadVIP (formerly Video Interaction Project) is an evidence-based parenting program promoting ERH. It adopts a relationship-based approach and uses real-time video feedback at pediatric health care visits to reinforce parenting strengths and enhance family resilience. During well-child visits from birth to 3 years, families meet with a PlayReadVIP coach who builds a caring, one-on-one relationship. In each session (approximately 25 minutes), the coach: (1) asks parents to reflect on their child's development while discussing anticipated developmental progress and potential parent-child activities; (2) provides parents with developmentally appropriate learning materials (eg, books or toys) that are subsequently used in a recorded 3-minute parent-child interaction (eg, shared reading and play); and (3) immediately watches the videotaped recording with the parents, highlighting their strengths in real time and suggesting additional opportunities for interaction.17 PlayReadVIP operates across 15 sites in 4 states and is extending globally in Brazil and Singapore.

PlayReadVIP has a significant impact on positive parenting and maternal mental health. For instance, PlayReadVIP was associated with increases in parents' reading, teaching, and verbal responsivity in Latinx and Black/African American populations[18,19] and those engaging in PlayReadVIP demonstrated reduced parenting stress, and depressive symptoms.[20,21] Increases in responsive parenting behaviors have been shown after a single visit, with additional increases following a second visit.[22]

PlayReadVIP has been shown to lead to enhanced mental health in children, including improved imitation/play, attention-reduced separation distress, and externalizing problems during the first 3 years,[23] with sustained reductions in hyperactivity[24] 1.5 years following program completion. PlayReadVIP also has impacts on children's cognitive, language, and early literacy development during toddlerhood and preschool years,[17] which operate directly and indirectly by means of enhancements in parental cognitive stimulation.[19,25,26] Importantly, given the mental health challenges and other social drivers of health among families served, ReadPlayVIP engagement is associated with increased engagement in clinical services delivered through home visiting.[27]

Family Nurture Intervention

Family Nurture Intervention (FNI) promotes emotional connection and sensitive caregiving behaviors between mothers and premature infants in neonatal intensive care (NICU) from birth through discharge. Using a relationship-based approach, nurse specialists are assigned to each family to facilitate intervention sessions (approximately 6 hours/week) that include scent cloth exchange, vocal soothing, emotion expression, eye contact, and skin-to-skin/clothed holding.[16,28] Extended family members are also engaged.[29]

FNI has been shown to promote mental health in children and their mothers. Studies have shown significant improvement in cognitive and language development, enhanced social relatedness, and reduced attention problems in preterm infants at 18 months.[28] Additionally, mothers participating in FNI demonstrated reduced depression and anxiety symptoms at 4 months corrected age.[30] Furthermore, mothers showed higher quality of maternal caregiving behavior, increased mother-infant face-to-face engagement at 4 months, and physical and psychological mother-infant coregulation in infancy and early childhood.[29–31]

Remote Delivery of Pediatric Mental Health Prevention Program

In response to the growing need for pediatric mental health services, there has been a notable trend toward the adoption of remote delivery approaches. Common methods include online platforms or applications, telehealth and video conferencing, social media, text messaging, and chat support, Web-based assessments, and surveys.[32,33] These innovative approaches have effectively addressed barriers that previously hindered family enrollment, including the high cost of traditional approaches, long waiting lists, childcare concerns, and transportation time. Moreover, they reduce stigma and offer flexibility and anonymity for participating families.[33,34] Remote delivery of these programs also facilitates population-based screening, enabling early detection of mental health issues in children and the potential use of data to personalize preventive interventions.[35]

Strongest Families Finland-Canada

Strongest Families Finland-Canada (SFFC) is a Finland-Canada collaborated, family-based prevention and treatment program for early childhood behavior problems. Families with 4-year-olds were randomly assigned to the Strongest Families Smart Web site (SFSW) group versus the educational control (EC). In the EC group, participants received access to a Web site containing positive parenting strategies and a call from a coach who provided additional positive parenting advice (in addition to standard care). In the SFFC group, participants were offered an online adaptation of the Strongest Families telephone-based program,[32] which includes online modules, exercises, and videos illustrating parenting skills and a weekly telephone call from a coach (licensed health care professional trained for the SWSF intervention).[33]

This Internet-and-telephone-assisted SFFC program has demonstrated effectiveness in enhancing child mental health outcomes. At the 12-month follow-up, children whose parents received SFSW exhibited improved internalizing, externalizing, and total behavior problems when compared with the EC group, as well as improved sleep, aggression, withdrawal, anxiety, emotional problems, and callousness. Finally, SFSW participants reported increased parenting skills[33] important for children's mental health.[36]

Dissemination of Prevention Strategies Across the Primary Care Community

Primary care providers are often the first point of contact for young children and their families. Training in innovative approaches can support a wide dissemination of prevention strategies. Reach Out and Read (ROR) is a key example. Founded in 1989 at Boston City Hospital, ROR is a national and global evidence-based pediatric literacy program supporting development in children aged 6 months to 5 years through a focus on sharing books.[37] ROR has several components: literacy-rich waiting rooms, anticipatory guidance, a new, developmentally appropriate book to take home, and modeled reading activities.[38,39] A key innovation of ROR is its capacity to train and involve primary care providers. That is, ROR's national center and affiliated networks have provided training for pediatric clinicians, family physicians, nurse practitioners, and physician assistants. To date, providers in over 4,000 clinics and practices have distributed more than 5.7 million new books and reading-aloud guidance to over 3.5 million children across all 50 states.[40] The large-scale involvement and training of health practitioners extends the reach of prevention efforts and have resulted in large impacts on parenting, optimal child outcomes in language development,[38,41] and reduced childhood toxic stress.[6]

Risk-Stratified Interventions Tailored to Families' Needs

Risk-stratified intervention, which matches families with programs of different intensity based on their risks and strengths, is an effective approach to ensure that children and their parents receive services that are tailored to their individual needs.[6,42] To allow for such matching, universal screening is offered as the first line of service to assess each family's challenges and needs.[42,43]

HealthySteps

HealthySteps (HS) uses a 3-tiered model to support ERH and child well-being from birth to 3 years.[44,45] In the first tier, universal services, such as screenings of child development and family needs and a child development support line, are offered to all families. In the second tier, families with mild-to-moderate risks for developmental problems, maternal depression, or social determinants of health receive short-term consultations about concerns for their child's development and/or parental well-being, referrals to services and resources, and information on positive parenting and early learning. In the third tier, families with the highest risks meet with a pediatric clinician and an HS specialist during their well-child visits, which provide educational information on positive parent-child interactions, child development, and maternal health.[44,45] As of 2023, HS was been implemented in over 260 sites across the United States and reached more than 405,000 children.[46]

Findings from quasi-experimental studies of HS showed that more intervention than control parents reported sharing picture books with their infants at least once a day at 2 to 4 months and 5 to 5.5 years.[47,48] Intervention parents were less likely than control parents to use harsh discipline (ie, spanking, slapping) at 30 to 33 months and 5 to 5.5 years, indicating a long-term impact of HS on parents' disciplinary practices.[47,48] Furthermore, a randomized control trial (RCT) found the effects of HS on observed maternal warmth and sensitivity, child secure attachment, and child behavior at 34 to 37 months.[49] Overall, findings indicate that HS has impacts on positive parenting behaviors that are known to promote children's mental health.[50,51]

Smart Beginnings

Smart Beginnings is a tiered model that combines PlayReadVIP and Family Check-Up (FCU) to promote school readiness and positive behavioral outcomes in children from birth to age 3.[19,25] PlayReadVIP is offered to all families in SB, while FCU, a secondary/tertiary home-visiting prevention program delivered by MSW (master of social work)-level family coaches,[52,53] is offered to families if they were found to have additional risk factors through screening (eg, maternal depression, low social support, difficult child temperament, child behavior problems) starting at 6 months. FCU includes 4 core components: (1) family assessment based on observation and interview, (2) relationship building and collaborative planning (get to know you), (3) strengths-based feedback, and (4) follow-up treatment sessions that build on parent-identified goals.[52]

Findings from an ongoing RCT demonstrate positive effects of SB on ERH and developmental outcomes in early childhood.[19,25,26,54] Specifically, SB moderated effects of perinatal maternal depression on child internalizing behaviors at 18 months, and families assigned to SB showed more positive parent-child interactions (eg, cognitive stimulation) at 6 and 24 months.[19,25].[54] These cognitively stimulating interactions at age 2 facilitated children's language and literacy at age 4.[26]

The Pittsburgh Study

The Pittsburgh Study (TPS) is a longitudinal, multi-cohort intervention designed to promote child health and thriving from birth to adolescence for all families living in Allegheny County, Pennsylvania.[55] A primary goal of TPS is to achieve population-level reach and impact through multiple family-friendly platforms, such as pediatric primary care, home visiting, Woman, Infants, and Children (WIC) clinics, family support and early learning centers, and libraries.[42,56] Families in TPS receive a short screening after enrollment to identify their strengths and challenges and then are offered two or more preventive programs that match their needs, including low-intensity programs (eg, text-based parent education) for families with few challenges, and moderate-to-high-intensity programs for families with more challenges. PlayReadVIP, FCU, and SB represent core components across multiple stratification levels. Quasi-experimental studies with the TPS early childhood cohort (0–5 years) will be conducted to examine the impacts of TPS from infancy to age 4 on early childhood outcomes, such as social-emotional development and positive parenting.[56] Preliminary findings suggest that TPS has successfully engaged families, especially those with higher risks, through population-level screening and provision of choice in parenting programs based on risk stratification (Krug CW, Mendelsohn AL, Wuerth J, et al. The Pittsburgh Study: a tiered model for supporting parents during early childhood. In revision.).

Team-Based Interventions Providing Family-Centered Care

An efficient method to expand the capacity of pediatric practices and increase the sustainability of child and family services is establishing an interdisciplinary care team, where pediatric providers and staff work together with intervention professionals.[57] PlayReadVIP and HS, as mentioned previously, both adopt a team-based care model by integrating an on-site child development professional into the well-child care team. Additionally, other interventions have taken a comprehensive approach to redesigning well-child visits by transferring providers' routine duties to intervention professionals and utilizing expertise from multiple sectors to provide family-centered care.

Parent-Focused Redesign for Encounters, Newborns to Toddlers

Parent-Focused Redesign for Encounters, Newborns to Toddlers (PARENT) adds a trained, master's-level parent coach (ie, health educator) to the pediatric care team, who provides families with children 0 to 3 years with anticipatory guidance, psychosocial screening and referral, and developmental/behavioral guidance and screening at each well-child visit.[58] Additionally, parents have access to a Web-based tool (the well-visit planner) for indicating their priorities for a visit, completing previsit screenings, and receiving a visit summary. Lastly, parents are sent biweekly text messages about anticipatory guidance, health education, and upcoming well-visits.[58] These intervention components build a well-rounded and tailored health care delivery system for individual families.[59]

Developmental Understanding and Legal Collaboration for Everyone

Developmental Understanding and Legal Collaboration for Everyone (DULCE) was developed to provide high-quality care for low-income families, families of color, and immigrants during the first 6 months of a child's life.[60] Similar to PARENT, it assigns each family a family specialist with postgraduate training in child development. The specialist attends every well-child visit for the first 6 months, conducts screening for health-related social needs, and offers developmental guidance. Additionally, the specialist meets weekly with an interdisciplinary team (a clinician, an early childhood system representative, a legal partner, and a clinic administrator) to review cases, identify community resources and legal services for families, and receive support on addressing unique family needs.[61,62]

RCTs of PARENT and DULCE showed more pediatric preventive care services, such as anticipatory guidance, well-child visits, and immunizations, at 6-month and 12-month follow-ups.[60,63] However, the impacts of these interventions on ERH and child development have not been assessed, thus calling for more research to understand their effectiveness related to child mental health.

Community-Based Interventions Building Resource Networks

A significant challenge faced by providers is connecting families with the resources that they need. To address this, pediatric preventive interventions have partnered with local communities to centralize resources and distribute information collectively to providers and families. For example, Help Me Grow (HMG), a model implemented across 28 states in the United States to facilitate early detection of developmental and behavioral problems, provides a centralized call center to support providers in effectively linking families with the right resources, and coordinating care.[64] Another example is Together Growing Strong (TGS), a place-based initiative in Sunset Park, Brooklyn, New York, a diverse neighborhood with a high poverty rate.[65] TGS integrates evidence-based programs in the community to improve services for families with young children. TGS includes 4 service components: (1) evidence-based programs in health care and schools, such as Reach Out and Stay Strong Essentials for New Mothers (ROSE),[66] PlayReadVIP, HS, ROR, and ParentCorps,[67] focused on child and maternal mental health, school readiness skills, and ERH; (2) digital messaging; (3) community workshops and events; and (4) support for clinicians and educators. A quasi-experimental study (the Children, Caregivers, and Community Study) involving 1350 families is underway to examine the impacts of TGS on child and family well-being from birth to school entry.[65] Through building local resource networks, HMG and TGS offer powerful platforms for pediatric clinicians to connect families with tailored resources and mental health service delivery.

DISCUSSION

Mental health challenges in early childhood are a risk factor for low educational attainment, risky behaviors, and poor mental and physical health during adolescence and adulthood.[4,5] ERH serves as a protective factor to mitigate the negative impacts of mental health issues among young children, highlighting an important point of intervention.[14] This article focused on 6 innovative approaches demonstrating recent research and practical efforts to more effectively engage families in pediatric preventive services to foster ERH and promote mental health in young children.

Among the interventions reviewed, several (ie, PlayReadVIP, FNI, SFFC, SB, and ROR) have demonstrated robust effects on early childhood mental health and key social-emotional antecedents, including reduced attention problems, and fewer externalizing and internalizing problems,[23,24,28,54,68] as well as enhancements in cognition, language, and literacy.[17,26,69] These interventions, together with HS, have shown improvements in positive parenting behaviors, such as cognitively stimulating interactions with children, mother-infant coregulation, maternal warmth and sensitivity, and more frequent parent-child book reading.[19,25,30,31,33,70,71] PlayReadVIP and FNI have also shown positive effects on parental mental health, such as reduced depression and parenting stress,[20,21,72,73] while SB buffered impacts of parental mental health on children.[54] For many other interventions, studies are underway to evaluate their benefits for child mental health (ie, TPS, PARENT, DULCE, HMG, and TGS).

Future Directions for Practice

Although the innovative approaches reviewed in this article can be impactful for improving pediatric mental health services and consequently mental health in early childhood, there are additional opportunities and directions that have received less attention and should also be considered. This includes promotion of initiatives that involve all family members, especially fathers. Pediatric prevention programs have predominantly focused on mothers, and there have been only limited efforts to engage fathers.[74] Fathers' mental health, involvement, and parenting behaviors play a significant role in the development of children's language, cognitive, and social-emotional skills in early childhood, as well as in managing stress in middle childhood.[51,75–78] Additionally, fathers' cognitively stimulating interactions with their young children have been found to support language and cognitive development, over and above the contribution of mothers.[79–82] Therefore, clinicians and future pediatric prevention programs should devote more efforts to including fathers and targeting their mental health and parenting as a way to promote child mental health.

Furthermore, the integration of management strategies for perinatal mental health such as depression within pediatric primary care settings should be prioritized to mitigate its impact on child behavioral and emotional difficulties.[83,84] Perinatal depression has a detrimental impact on mothers' caregiving practices (eg, breastfeeding), mothers' and fathers' parenting behaviors (eg, reading to their child), family functioning, and child mental health.[85–87] Although existing interventions involving pregnant women, such as ROSE, have demonstrated positive impacts on perinatal depression,[66] there is a pressing need for pediatric practices to incorporate services and treatments for perinatal depression.[83] Some of the recommended approaches by the American Academy of Pediatrics (AAP) share key elements with the pediatric mental health prevention programs discussed in this article, such as team-based services by coordinating care between pediatric medical homes and prenatal providers for perinatally depressed women, universal screening for postpartum depression as a first line of services offered during well-child visits, community-based programs with resource networks to connect mothers with appropriate services, and relationship-based intervention to support positive parent-child relationships.[83] By adopting these strategies, pediatric clinics can play a pivotal role in supporting not just the health of the child but the well-being of the entire family.

SUMMARY

Pediatric primary care is an ideal platform for early prevention, because programs can leverage the existing infrastructure and pediatrician-parent relationship to reduce implementation costs, enhance uptake, and utilize the frequent well-child visits during early childhood to achieve dose and impact. The reviewed innovative approaches demonstrate strong potential to foster child mental health and present opportunities to overcome some significant challenges in pediatric preventive care by nourishing trusting relationships between families and child development professionals, accommodating remote delivery, disseminating training to health professionals, offering universal screening and tailored services, engaging interdisciplinary expertise, and building centralized resources. Moving forward, more research is needed to systematically assess the direct and indirect mechanisms through which pediatric primary care interventions promote child mental health and to evaluate the roles of fathers and maternal mental health in pediatric prevention programs.

CLINICS CARE POINTS

- Promote early relational health as an opportunity for supporting children's mental health.
- Embrace innovative strategies such as relationship-based approaches, remote delivery, dissemination of prevention strategies, risk-stratified interventions, team-based interventions, and community-based interventions to actively involve families in preventive service and promote mental health in young children.
- Involve fathers and implement integrative strategies addressing perinatal maternal mental health for better prevention outcomes for children's mental health.

DISCLOSURE

The authors have nothing to disclose.

FUNDING

We would like to thank the funders for supporting the authors' current research and intervention work, including the National Institutes of Health/National Institute of Child Health and Human Development (R01 HD047740 01–09 and R01 HD076390 01–02), the Tiger Foundation, the Marks Family Foundation, Children of Bellevue, Inc., KiDS of NYU Foundation, Inc., and City's First Readers. We would also like to thank the parents and children who have participated in our programs and research studies.

REFERENCES

1. Brookman RR. Mental health disorders in adolescents. Obstet Gynecol 2017; 130(1):247–8.
2. Merikangas K, He J Ping, Burstein M, et al. Lifetime prevalence of mental disorders in us adolescents: results from the national comorbidity study-adolescent supplement (NCS-A). J Am Acad Child Adolesc Psychiatr 2010;49(10):980–9.
3. Robinson LR, Holbrook JR, Bitsko RH, et al. Differences in health care, family, and community factors associated with mental, behavioral, and developmental disorders among children aged 2-8 years in rural and Urban Areas - United States, 2011-2012. MMWR Surveillance Summaries 2017;66(8):1–11.

4. Otto C, Reiss F, Voss C, et al. Mental health and well-being from childhood to adulthood: design, methods and results of the 11-year follow-up of the BELLA study. Eur Child Adolesc Psychiatr 2021;30(10):1559–77.
5. Younger DS. Epidemiology of childhood mental illness: a review of US surveillance data and the literature. World J Neurosci 2017;07(01):48–54.
6. Garner A, Yogman M, Committee on Psychosocial Aspects of Child and Family Health, Section on Developmental and Behavioral Pediatrics Coec. Preventing childhood toxic stress: partnering with families and communities to promote relational health. Am Acad Pediatr 2021;148(2). Available at: http://publications.aap.org/pediatrics/article-pdf/148/2/e2021052582/1440326/peds_2021052582.pdf.
7. World Health Organization. The importance of caregiver-child interactions for the survival and healthy development of young children. World Health Organization. Available at: https://www.who.int/publications/i/item/924159134X. (Accessed January 13 2024).
8. Frosch CA, Schoppe-Sullivan SJ, O'Banion DD. Parenting and child development: a relational health perspective. Am J Lifestyle Med 2021;15(1):45–59.
9. Rojas LM, Bahamón M, Wagstaff R, et al. Evidence-based prevention programs targeting youth mental and behavioral health in primary care: a systematic review. Prev Med 2019;120:85–99.
10. Kolko D, Perrin E. The integration of behavioral health interventions in children's health care: services, science, and suggestions. J Clin Child Adolesc Psychol 2014;43(2):216–28.
11. Wissow LS, Van Ginneken N, Chandna J, et al. Integrating children's mental health into primary care Lawrence. Pediatr Clin 2016;63(1):97–113.
12. Noble KG, Houston SM, Brito NH, et al. Family income, parental education and brain structure in children and adolescents. Nat Neurosci 2015;18(5):773–8.
13. Browne DT, Wade M, May SS, et al. Children's mental health problems during the initial emergence of COVID-19. Can Psychol 2021;62(1):65–72.
14. Li J., Ramirez T., Early relational health: A review of research, principles, and perspectives, The Burke Foundation, 2023. Available at: https://burkefoundation.org/burke-portfolio/reports/early-relational-health-a-review-of-research-principles-and-perspectives/. (Accessed August 13, 2024).
15. Heffron MC. Clarifying concepts of infant mental health- promotion, relationship-based preventive intervention, and treatment. Infants Young Child 2000;12(4):14–21.
16. Hane AA, Myers MM, Hofer MA, et al. Family nurture intervention improves the quality of maternal caregiving in the neonatal intensive care unit: evidence from a randomized controlled trial. J Dev Behav Pediatr 2015;36(3):188–96.
17. Mendelsohn AL, Valdez PT, Flynn V, et al. Use of videotaped interactions during pediatric well-child care: impact at 33 months on parenting and on child development. J Dev Behav Pediatr 2007;28(3):206–12.
18. Mendelsohn AL, Huberman HS, Berkule SB, et al. Primary care strategies for promoting parent-child interactions and school readiness in at-risk families: the Bellevue Project for Early Language, Literacy, and Education Success. Arch Pediatr Adolesc Med 2011;165(1):33–41.
19. Roby E, Miller EB, Shaw DS, et al. Improving parent-child interactions in pediatric health care: a two-site randomized controlled trial. Pediatrics 2021;147(3). https://doi.org/10.1542/PEDS.2020-1799.
20. Cates CB, Weisleder A, Dreyer BP, et al. Leveraging healthcare to promote responsive parenting: impacts of the video interaction project on parenting stress. J Child Fam Stud 2016;25(3):827–35.

21. Berkule SB, Cates CB, Dreyer BP, et al. Reducing maternal depressive symptoms through promotion of parenting in pediatric primary care. Clin Pediatr (Phila). 2014;53(5):460–9.
22. Piccolo LR, Roby E, Canfield CF, et al. Supporting responsive parenting in real-world implementation: minimal effective dose of the Video Interaction Project. Pediatr Res 2023;(June;1–6. https://doi.org/10.1038/s41390-023-02916-4.
23. Weisleder A, Cates CB, Dreyer BP, et al. Promotion of positive parenting and prevention of socioemotional disparities. Pediatrics 2016;137(2). https://doi.org/10.1542/peds.2015-3239.
24. Mendelsohn AL, Brockmeyer CC, Weisleder A, et al. Reading aloud, play , and social-emotional development 2018;141(5):e20173393.
25. Miller EB, Roby E, Zhang Y, et al. Promoting cognitive stimulation in parents across infancy and toddlerhood: a randomized clinical trial. J Pediatr 2023;255: 159–65.e4.
26. Miller EB, Canfield CF, Roby E, et al. Enhancing early language and literacy skills for racial/ethnic minority children with low incomes through a randomized clinical trial: The mediating role of cognitively stimulating parent–child interactions. Child Dev 2023;1–14. https://doi.org/10.1111/cdev.14064.
27. Canfield CF, Miller EB, Zhang Y, et al. Tiered universal and targeted early childhood interventions: enhancing attendance across families with varying needs. Early Child Res Q 2023;63(January):362–9.
28. Welch MG, Firestein MR, Austin J, et al. Family nurture intervention in the neonatal intensive care unit improves social-relatedness, attention, and neurodevelopment of preterm infants at 18 months in a randomized controlled trial. JCPP (J Child Psychol Psychiatry) 2015;56(11):1202–11.
29. Welch MG, Hofer MA, Brunelli SA, et al. Family nurture intervention (FNI): methods and treatment protocol of a randomized controlled trial in the NICU. BMC Pediatr 2012;12:1–17.
30. Beebe B, Myers MM, Lange A, et al. Family nurture intervention for preterm infants facilitates positive mother–infant face-to-face engagement at 4 months. Dev Psychol 2018;54(11):2016–31.
31. Welch MG, Barone JL, Porges SW, et al. Family nurture intervention in the NICU increases autonomic regulation in mothers and children at 4-5 years of age: Follow-up results from a randomized controlled trial. PLoS One 2020;15(8 August):1–19.
32. McGrath PJ, Lingley-Pottie P, Thurston C, et al. Telephone-based mental health interventions for child disruptive behavior or anxiety disorders: randomized trials and overall analysis. Pscychol Res Behav Manag 2011;50:1162–72.
33. Sourander A, McGrath PJ, Ristkari T, et al. Internet-assisted parent training intervention for disruptive behavior in 4-year-old children: a randomized clinical trial. JAMA Psychiatr 2016;73(4):378–87.
34. McGrath P, Sourander A, Lingley-Pottie P, et al. Remote population-based intervention for disruptive behavior at age four: study protocol for a randomized trial of Internet-assisted parent training (Strongest Families Finland-Canada). BMC Publ Health 2013;13(985). https://doi.org/10.1186/2046-1682-4-13.
35. Bergin AD, Vallejos EP, Davies EB, et al. Preventive digital mental health interventions for children and young people: a review of the design and reporting of research. NPJ Digit Med 2020;3(1). https://doi.org/10.1038/s41746-020-00339-7.
36. Phelan RF, Howe DJ, Cashman EL, et al. Enhancing parenting skills for parents with mental illness: the Mental Health Positive Parenting Program. Med J Aust 2013;199(3):S30–3.

37. Mendelsohn AL. Promoting language and literacy through reading aloud: The role of the pediatrician. Curr Probl Pediatr Adolesc Health Care 2002;32(6): 188–202.
38. Jimenez ME, Uthirasamy N, Hemler JR, et al. Maximizing the impact of reach out and read literacy promotion: anticipatory guidance and modeling. Pediatr Res 2023;(August;1–5. https://doi.org/10.1038/s41390-023-02945-z.
39. Klass P, Dreyer BP, Mendelsohn AL. Reach out and read: literacy promotion in pediatric primary care. Adv Pediatr 2009;56:11–27.
40. Zuckerman B, Khandekar A. Reach out and read: evidence-based approach to promoting early child development. Curr Opin Pediatr 2010;22(4):539–44.
41. Garbe CM, Bond SL, Boulware C, et al. The effect of exposure to reach out and read on shared reading behaviors. Acad Pediatr 2023;23(8):1598–604.
42. Shaw DS, Mendelsohn AL, Morris PA. Reducing poverty-related disparities in child development and school readiness: the smart beginnings tiered prevention strategy that combines pediatric primary care with home visiting. Clin Child Fam Psychol Rev 2021;24(4):669–83.
43. Wissow LS, Brown J, Fothergill KE, et al. Universal mental health screening in pediatric primary care: a systematic review. J Am Acad Child Adolesc Psychiatry 2013;52(11):1134–47.e23.
44. Minkovitz C, Strobino D, Hughart N, et al, Healthy Steps Evaluation Team. Early effects of the healthy steps for young children program. Arch Pediatr Adolesc Med 2001;155. https://doi.org/10.1001/archpedi.155.4.470.
45. Valado T, Tracey J, Goldfinger J, et al. HealthySteps: transforming the promise of pediatric Care. Future of Children 2019;29(1):99–122.
46. HealthySteps. HealthySteps Our Impact. 2023. Available at: https://www.healthysteps.org/our-impact/. [Accessed 26 March 2024].
47. Minkovitz CS, Strobino D, Mistry KB, et al. Healthy steps for young children: Sustained results at 5.5 years. Pediatrics 2007;120(3). https://doi.org/10.1542/peds.2006-1205.
48. Minkovitz CS, Hughart N, Strobino D, et al. A practice-based intervention to enhance quality of care in the first 3 years of life: the Healthy Steps for Young Children Program. JAMA 2003;290(23):3081–91.
49. Caughy MOB, Huang KY, Miller T, et al. The effects of the Healthy Steps for Young Children Program: results from observations of parenting and child development. Early Child Res Q 2004;19(4):611–30.
50. Fagan J, Cabrera N. Trajectories of low-income mothers' and fathers' engagement in learning activities and child socioemotional skills in middle childhood. Soc Dev 2023;32(2):672–89.
51. Tamis-LeMonda CS, Briggs RD, McClowry SG, et al. Maternal control and sensitivity, child gender, and maternal education in relation to children's behavioral outcomes in African American families. J Appl Dev Psychol 2009;30(3):321–31.
52. Shaw DS, Supplee L, Dishion TJ, et al. Randomized trial of a family-centered approach to the prevention of early conduct problems: 2-Year effects of the family check-up in early childhood. J Consult Clin Psychol 2006;74(1):1–9.
53. Shaw DS, Galán CA, Lemery-Chalfant K, et al. Trajectories and predictors of children's early-starting conduct problems: child, family, genetic, and intervention effects. Dev Psychopathol 2019;31(5):1911–21.
54. Canfield CF, Miller EB, Taraban L, et al. Impacts of a tiered intervention on child internalizing and externalizing behavior in the context of maternal depression. Dev Psychopathol 2023. https://doi.org/10.1017/S0954579423001475.

55. Dermody TS, Ettinger A, Savage Friedman F, et al. The Pittsburgh Study: learning with communities about child health and thriving. Health Equity 2022;6(1): 338–44.
56. Roby E, Shaw DS, Morris P, et al. Pediatric primary care and partnerships across sectors to promote early child development. Acad Pediatr 2021;21(2):228–35.
57. Turchi RM, Antonelli RC, Norwood KW, et al. Patient- and family-centered care coordination: a framework for integrating care for children and youth across multiple systems. Pediatrics 2014;133(5). https://doi.org/10.1542/peds.2014-0318.
58. Coker TR, Chacon S, Elliott MN, et al. A parent coach model for well-child care among low-income children: a randomized controlled trial. Pediatrics 2016; 137(3):e20153013.
59. Mimila NA, Chung PJ, Elliott MN, et al. Well-child care redesign: a mixed methods analysis of parent experiences in the PARENT trial. Acad Pediatr 2017;17(7): 747–54.
60. Sege R, Preer G, Morton SJ, et al. Medical-legal strategies to improve infant health care: a randomized trial. Pediatrics 2015;136(1):97–106.
61. Arbour MC, Fico P, Atwood S, et al. Benefits of a universal intervention in pediatric medical homes to identify and address health-related social needs: an observational Cohort Study. Acad Pediatr 2022;22(8):1328–37.
62. Arbour MC, Floyd B, Morton S, et al. Cross-sector approach expands screening and addresses health-related social needs in primary care. Pediatrics 2021; 148(5). https://doi.org/10.1542/peds.2021-050152.
63. Coker TR, Liljenquist K, Lowry SJ, et al. Community health workers in early childhood well-child care for medicaid-insured children: a randomized clinical trial. JAMA 2023;329(20):1757–67.
64. Help Me Grow promotes optimal child development by enhancing protective factors successfully addressing the needs of at-risk children, Available at: http://www.cssp.org/reform/strengthening-families/basic-one-pagers/Strengthening-Families-Protective-Factors.pdf. (Accessed January 22 2024).
65. Miller EB, Canfield CF, Barajas-Gonzalez RG, et al. The Children, Caregivers, and Community (C3) study of together growing strong: a protocol for an observational, place-based initiative in Sunset Park, Brooklyn. PLoS One 2023;18(9 September). https://doi.org/10.1371/journal.pone.0290985.
66. Zlotnick C, Tzilos G, Miller I, et al. Randomized controlled trial to prevent postpartum depression in mothers on public assistance. J Affect Disord 2016;189: 263–8.
67. Miller Brotman L, Dawson-McClure S, Kamboukos D, et al. Effects of Parentcorps in prekindergarten on child mental health and academic performance follow-up of a randomized clinical trial through 8 years of age. JAMA Pediatr 2016; 170(12):1149–55.
68. Achenbach TM, Ruffle TM. The child behavior checklist and related forms for assessing behavioral/emotional problems and competencies. Pediatr Rev 2000; 21(8):265–71.
69. High PC, LaGasse L, Becker S, et al. Literacy promotion in primary care pediatrics: Can we make a difference? Pediatrics 2000;105(4 II):927–34.
70. Cates CB, Weisleder A, Berkule Johnson S, et al. Enhancing parent talk, reading, and play in primary care: sustained impacts of the video interaction project. J Pediatr 2018;199:49–56.e1.
71. Canfield CF, Seery A, Weisleder A, et al. Encouraging parent–child book sharing: potential additive benefits of literacy promotion in health care and the community. Early Child Res Q 2020;50:221–9.

72. Welch MG, Halperin MS, Austin J, et al. Depression and anxiety symptoms of mothers of preterm infants are decreased at 4 months corrected age with Family Nurture Intervention in the NICU. Arch Womens Ment Health 2016;19(1):51–61.
73. Weisleder A, Cates CB, Harding JF, et al. Links between shared reading and play, parent psychosocial functioning, and child behavior: evidence from a randomized controlled trial. J Pediatr 2019;213:187–95.e1.
74. Izett E, Rooney R, Prescott SL, et al. Prevention of mental health difficulties for children aged 0–3 years: a review. Front Psychol 2021;11. https://doi.org/10.3389/fpsyg.2020.500361.
75. Cabrera NJ, Tamis-Lemonda CS, Bradley RH, et al. Fatherhood in the twenty-first century. Child Dev 2000;71(1):127–36.
76. Fitzgerald HE, Robinson LR, Cabrera N, et al. Fathers and families: risk and resilience. an introduction. Advers Resil Sci 2021;2(2):63–9.
77. Paulson JF, Keefe HA, Leiferman JA. Early parental depression and child language development. JCPP (J Child Psychol Psychiatry) 2009;50(3):254–62.
78. Roby E, Piccolo LR, Gutierrez J, et al. Father involvement in infancy predicts behavior and response to chronic stress in middle childhood in a low-income Latinx sample. Dev Psychobiol 2021;63(5):1449–65.
79. Cox MJ, Paley B. Understanding families as systems. Curr Dir Psychol Sci 2003;12(5):193–6.
80. Cabrera NJ, Jeong Moon U, Fagan J, et al. Cognitive stimulation at home and in child care and children's preacademic skills in two-parent families. Child Dev 2020;91(5):1709–17.
81. Chen Y, Cabrera NJ, Reich SM. Mother-child and father-child "serve and return" interactions at 9 months: associations with children's language skills at 18 and 24 months. Infant Behav Dev 2023;73. https://doi.org/10.1016/j.infbeh.2023.101894.
82. Tamis-LeMonda CS, Shannon JD, Cabrera NJ, et al. Fathers and mothers at play with their 2- and 3-year-olds: contributions to language and cognitive development. Child Dev 2004;75(6):1806–20.
83. Earls MF, Yogman MW, Mattson G, et al. Incorporating recognition and management of perinatal depression into pediatric practice. Pediatrics 2019;143(1):e20183259.
84. Olin SCS, Kerker B, Stein REK, et al. Can postpartum depression be managed in pediatric primary care? J Womens Health 2016;25(4):381–90.
85. Fentz HN, Nygaard K, Simonsen M, et al. The influence of depressive symptoms on parenting: examining longitudinal dyadic spillover and crossover processes during the transition to parenthood. J Fam Issues 2023;44(2):455–74.
86. Field T. Postpartum depression effects on early interactions, parenting, and safety practices: a review. Infant Behav Dev 2010;33(1):1–6.
88. Muzik M, Borovska S. Perinatal depression: implications for child mental health perinatal depression: prevalence and treatment seeking. Ment Health Fam Med 2010;7:239–47.

Trauma-Informed Strategies in Pediatric Primary Care

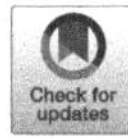

Heather Forkey, MD[a,*], Jessica Griffin, PsyD[b]

KEYWORDS

• Trauma-informed care • Child trauma • Trauma • Trauma-focused treatment
• Affiliate response • Stress response

KEY POINTS

- Trauma-informed care (TIC) applies the science of the stress response, particularly the critical role of the affiliate response.
- TIC begins with engagement that promotes safety.
- Surveillance and screening for both exposures and symptoms can guide diagnosis and treatment. Adverse Childhood Experiences screening has value in measuring the exposures of communities but is not clinically useful.
- Treatment begins with validating the patient's experience, providing both psychoeducation and strategies to calm the stress response.
- There are multiple evidence-based trauma therapies that can be provided to youth to reduce symptoms and improve protective factors and outcomes for youth and families.

BACKGROUND

Trauma was first introduced as a diagnostic and statistical manual of mental disorders (DSM) diagnosis in 1980 in explaining the responses of those who had lived through wartime traumas.[1] Prior to that trauma was described by patient and trauma characteristics, including "soldier's heart," "nostalgia," "battle fatigue," or "shell shock"; these terms reflected the perception that the reactions were due to a character flaw in the patient. Since then, our understanding of trauma, and the particularly profound effect of traumas that occur in childhood, as well as its treatment has evolved considerably. The Adverse Childhood Experiences (ACE) study, published in 1998, was one of the first large-scale studies to identify the commonality of early childhood adversity and the lifelong consequences of early relational trauma (or trauma that happens in the

[a] Department of Pediatrics, UMass Chan Medical School, UMass Memorial Children's Medical Center, 55 Lake Avenue North, Benedict Building A2-201, Worcester, MA 01655, USA; [b] Lifeline for Kids, Department of Psychiatry, UMass Chan Medical School, 55 Lake Avenue, North Worcester, MA 01655, USA
* Corresponding author.
E-mail address: Heather.Forkey@umassmemorial.org
Twitter: @TheDrJessica (J.G.)

Pediatr Clin N Am 71 (2024) 1101–1117
https://doi.org/10.1016/j.pcl.2024.07.016 pediatric.theclinics.com
0031-3955/24/

context of a caregiving relationship).[2] The ACE study demonstrated that for adults who had experienced 1 of 10 household adversities (emotional, physical or sexual abuse, physical or emotional neglect, domestic violence, caregiver loss due to incarceration or divorce, caregiver impairment due to substance use, or mental illness), there were associations with poorer health outcomes in adulthood. In the 20 years since its publication, significant advancements in neurophysiology, endocrinology, and epidemiology have helped to elucidate how early adversities (including, but not limited to, those in the original ACE study) become biologically embedded leading not only to mental health consequences but also to effects on development, educational attainment, physical health, and longevity.[3–11]

We have learned that early relational trauma causes its long-term effects through alterations of the stress response.[4,6,12] Humans have evolved over millions of years to have a few ways of managing stressors or threats. Most are familiar with the stress responses of fight (aggressive confrontation) or flight (running away or avoidance) or freeze (do nothing and hope the stressor moves past you). Yet, for humans in a setting of predatory threat, these stress responses have limitations. Humans are relatively large and likely to be spotted if we freeze. Without claws, an inability to hide under water, and a running speed slower than most of the animals, we needed to outpace to survive, fight or flight also have limited benefit. In fact, survival favored seeking the support of other humans when we felt the most threatened—to find food, fight off predators, and to raise our young.[13–15]

This last stress response is called the affiliate response or "tend and befriend."[14,16] The hormone oxytocin drives humans to identify if there are others close by to seek support from and provide support to when conditions allow. Oxytocin drives our efforts to seek support from others, and when we are successful, to benefit from that safety and calming of stress hormones (eg, decreases cortisol, adrenaline, and norepinephrine).[17–20] And use of the affiliate response is not a decision, but an appetitive need.[14]

The affiliate response is how children primarily seek to address their needs and address most stressors in their environment. The cry of the infant, the whining of the toddler, and the clinginess of a child indicate that they are seeking the affiliate support of the caregiver. Fortunately, the oxytocin hormone promotes brain changes in caregivers too, which allow them to attune to children, to orient to their needs and to find joy (through oxytocin-mediated effects of reward pathways) in the interactions with their children. In this way, humans create dyadic, mutually regulated systems of stress relief through safe, stable, nurturing relationships (SSNRs).[13,18,19] This has a great evolutionary advantage—the immature undeveloped brains of children are regulated and can develop with the external regulation of the caregiver developed brain.[13,18] And as we grow, our unique ability to band together under stress and work toward common goals gives us an advantage. This is the underpinning of why humans need SSNRs.

In fact, all children experience stress and adversity at some point in life, but when it is managed within the context of nurturing relationships, such events can be weathered and even used for growth. What early relational trauma represents is the condition by which SSNRs are unavailable or insufficient, and our neurobiological stress response shunts from affiliative to the fight–flight–freeze pathway. A person whose body is in fight–flight–freeze mode experiences a cascade of stress hormones and biological processes in response. If the stress is prolonged, frequent, or severe and there is a marked imbalance between stressors and protective factors, "toxic stress" can result.[11] Toxic stress is the physiologic effect of prolonged activation of the stress hormones cortisol and norepinephrine. Thus, the toxic stress response results from 2 components: (1) the effect of the adverse event(s) and (2) the insufficiency of protective relationships.[11,21]

With this underlying physiology in mind, the goals of TIC are to "assess, recognize and respond to the effects of traumatic experiences on children, caregivers and health care providers."[22,23] Unfortunately, many of the descriptions of TIC focus on important principles of safety, transparency and trustworthiness, empowerment voice and choice, peer support, collaboration and mutuality, and cultural humility, which are critical underpinnings, but not specific clinical guidance.[24] In response to a perceived lack of clinical strategy, some clinicians have turned to employing a version of the ACE questionnaire research tool used by Anda and Filetti in clinical settings.[2] As we will explain, while providing our patients with an ACE score may give the appearance of diagnostic certainty, an ACE score has validity in populations, but no clinical validity at the individual patient level.[25–27] Indeed, trauma-informed care is about relationships and is rooted in the affiliate stress response. It is about applying empathy and engagement, connecting, collaborating, and meeting the reality of our patients' lives. Thus, *instead of just summing the suffering, pediatric trauma-informed care builds the buffering of relational health.*

CLINICAL STRATEGIES

Trauma-informed care does not require a new approach to pediatric care but allows us to do what we already do with a trauma lens. Trauma-informed care includes all the steps used in day-to-day pediatric care.[28] They include

1. *Preparation and training*—learning about the epidemiology and physiology of trauma and the signs and symptoms of trauma reactions. For those working with children, this can include a 2 generation approach, considering how trauma may impact children, but also how caregivers may have experienced early trauma and how that will impact how they parent and respond to their child. It involves promoting resilience and evaluating how trauma may play a part in all types of pediatric visits.
2. *Engagement*—how to set the stage for TIC, creating a safe experience for children and families as we raise and respond to trauma.
3. *Surveillance and screening*—what tools will be used to gather information about what a child has experienced and how that is impacting their behavior and development.
4. *Diagnosis*—what the spectrum of trauma is, how it gets named and explained to families.
5. *Treatment*—both in office or hospital and what referrals need to be made. For a small subset of children, medication may need to be considered.

In "Background" section, we covered some of that preparation and training and we encourage you to continue that process. Next we will highlight tips for engagement, surveillance and screening, diagnosis, and treatment.

Engagement

To provide trauma-informed care, we first need to connect with families in nonthreatening, welcoming ways. Without connection, trust, and a sense of safety in the patient–pediatrician relationship, interventions may be misinformed, misguided, or fail. Neuroception is a term for the human capacity to perceive danger constantly and rapidly through all the senses and through social cues.[29] That is why engagement strategies that create a sense of safety and trust are critical to a trauma-informed response. When greeting patients, it is important to pay attention to our tone and demeanor—using welcoming, friendly language addressing everyone in the room (child and caregivers) and asking open-ended questions (eg, how are you? What brings you in today?). Even if the provider does not agree, it is important to focus on the caregiver's and patient's initial concern. Attuned and active listening is strongly encouraged. Basic rules for engagement include talking in a level that is appropriate for their age, using lay language and avoiding overly complex terms or explaining complex terms when necessary, reflecting back to them using the family's language or terminology, maintaining eye contact when culturally appropriate, communicating clearly, slowly, and directly, asking what questions they may have and checking in about what has worked for the family and what supports they have in place.

Professionals can be encouraged to use motivational interviewing, which involves expressing empathy for families' positions while not arguing with them or telling them what to do and helping them to resolve discrepancies and support their own self-efficacy and decision-making. Another set of engagement strategies, "LACE" a mnemonic adapted from Baylin and Hughes[30] can be used to connect with families and help them feel more understood. LACE includes lightheartedness (use gentle tone and demeanor, humor, and higher pitched voice), acceptance (using a nonjudgmental and respectful approach with families), curiosity (ask open-ended questions to understand their concerns or the meaning of certain behaviors), and empathy (normalize their response to trauma, validate strong emotions, and help them manage distress).

Lastly, to further engagement, psychoeducation (described later) allows the physician to help relieve some of the family's distress, which can increase their engagement in services. By helping families understand that it is not about what is wrong with their child but what has happened to their child and normalizing the response the child and caregivers had to their traumatic experiences, this trauma-informed shift can increase validation and understanding felt by families.

Surveillance and Screening

After we have engaged with the patient and family, we are in a better position to obtain more information about exposure and symptoms using surveillance and screening. In most instances, more information is needed to determine if trauma is the cause of the signs or symptoms that bring the child to care. In fact, if we do not ask about trauma, families may not bring it up. Yet an *important principle is that if we hear about trauma symptoms, we should consider trauma exposure, and if we hear about trauma exposure, we should investigate for trauma symptoms.* As a first step, surveillance, or the use of open-ended questions can begin the conversation about trauma as a cause and provide information about the need to gather more information.[28] Simple questions that are useful include

- Has anything scary or upsetting happened recently or since your last visit?
- Has anyone come or gone from the household lately?

Screening is a much more thorough and accurate way to gather information about exposure and symptoms. Some tools include question about potential trauma exposure and social drivers of health (Survey of Well-being of Young Children [SWYC], Safe Environment for Every Kid [SEEK]).[31,32] But, the most effective tools are those that combine questions about exposure to adverse events and traumatic stress symptoms. As noted earlier, current research does not support screening for ACEs alone, as these tools have validity in populations, but are not predictive of individual outcomes.[26] Robert Anda, one of the authors of the original ACE study has written, "the ACE questionnaire was designed to research—not screen—the relationship between childhood adversities and health and social outcomes."[27]

Part of screening includes explaining the purpose and use of the tool and process. Points to include are why the screening is being done, how the results will be used and stored, and what are the benefits to the child and family. Sharing that confidentiality will be kept unless the child indicates harm to themselves or others can help, especially with families who have experienced trauma. Before screening, primary care providers should have strategies in place to address safety including how to report to child protective services when needed and how to address suicidal concerns if those are identified.

Screening may be handled differently depending on the age and developmental stage of the child and on the availability of a caregiver to report on that child's exposure and symptoms. Caregivers are usually asked to report on symptoms for young children, but this is not always accurate or even possible, as children new to foster care may not come to appointments with a caregiver who is aware of this information, and for young children, "trauma symptoms" may be hard to assess. General behavioral or developmental screening can provide some insight.

For older children, it is usually appropriate to screen for trauma symptoms using the tools discussed later, which include questions about exposure and symptoms. Using these alone or pairing these tools with other brief and widely available tools for issues such as anxiety and depression can help to distinguish if overlapping symptoms are the result of trauma.[33] These tools can identify children with traumatic stress symptoms who may benefit from further evaluation and evidence-based trauma therapy. Traumatic stress screening may be implemented at well child visits or may be used only when concerns are raised, such as at pediatric behavioral health visits (eg, concerns for attention deficit hyperactivity disorder [ADHD], depression, anxiety, and behavior problems) or when a patient reports a potentially traumatic event. These tools may also be used to monitor trauma symptoms.

Available tools based on the DSM-5 criteria for PTSD include

- Child and Adolescent Trauma Screen is a freely accessible screening instrument (validated; 40 questions; ages 7–17 years)[34];
- Child Trauma Screen (CTS) is a brief, freely accessible screening instrument (validated; 10 questions; ages 6–17 years, with ages 3–6 years in development)[35];
- Pediatric Traumatic Stress Screening Tool is a brief, freely accessible screening instrument (15 questions, which includes the University of California, Los Angeles (UCLA) Brief Screen for Trauma and PTSD; ages 6–10 years, 11–18 years)[33];
- UCLA Brief Screen for Trauma and PTSD is a brief screening instrument, requires licensing agreement for use (validated; 11 questions; ages >6 years)[36]; and
- Child PTSD Symptom Scale for DSM-5 is a freely accessible screening instrument (validated; 27 items, ages 8–18 years).[37,38]

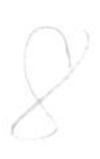

After screening, it is important to share the results with the child and caregivers and explain how the results inform the next steps. Normalizing, or explaining that the child's feelings are normal and expected given the events that have happened is an important follow-up to screening. For example, "When you filled out the form, you checked the question about having a lot of trouble with nightmares, and with thinking about the event when it just pops into your head. Those are symptoms we often hear about after an accident like the one you mentioned. In fact, it tells us your brain is trying to keep you safe. Even though it is a normal response to the accident, it is really hard to have nightmares and those thoughts popping into your head anytime, so we'd like to refer you to a therapist that specializes in helping people who have been through upsetting or scary things and have the same kinds of reactions."

Diagnosis

Discriminating trauma diagnoses can be challenging. Medical providers may encounter children with a wide range of symptoms and presentations resulting from trauma. This is due to factors that include

- Symptoms are the result not just of the traumatic exposure, but trauma factors of timing, frequency, and intensity; child factors including age, developmental stage, and genetic vulnerability; and most especially, the supports or emotional buffers in a child's life.
- Symptoms from can evolve over time, either worsening or resolving depending on factors noted earlier.
- Symptoms can present in various domains of function from sleep, appetite, and toileting (eg, overeating, insomnia, constipation, or enuresis) to development and school functioning (eg, delays in developmental milestones, poor attention, and school avoidance) to somatic concerns (eg, headache and stomach-ache) and immune system function (eg, inflammatory upregulation and infection susceptibility).[28]
- Symptoms overlap with other diagnoses such as ADHD, depression, anxiety, and autism spectrum disorder. In fact, it has been proposed that trauma represents a different "ecophenotype" of common disorders with similar presentations but unique trajectories and treatment response patterns.[39]
- Children may have conditions that are comorbid with trauma, as the biological and environmental conditions that lead to ADHD, anxiety, depression, fetal alcohol disorder, or developmental and learning issues, frequently are present in the setting of childhood trauma.
- Adding to confusion in pediatrics is the fact that trauma diagnoses have not traditionally been a part of training and represent a "GAP" in pediatric training. GAP is also an acronym for the most common trauma diagnoses.
- Grief—prolonged grief disorder
- Adjustment—adjustment disorder
- PTSD—posttraumatic stress disorder
- Traumatic events that involve severe early victimization without caregiver support such that there is disruption of the protective caregiving bond can result in symptoms that extend into multiple domains of functioning. This has been named developmental trauma disorder or complex trauma, and though used and considered distinct from posttraumatic stress disorder by trauma experts, it is not yet a part of the DSM. The areas impacted and symptoms noted include those impacted by PTSD plus disorders of self-organization including affect dysregulation, negative self-concept, and disturbances in relationships. Many of these symptoms overlap with symptoms of oppositional defiant disorder, anxiety, depression, conduct disorder, and disruptive mood dysregulation disorder, further confounding diagnosis.[40,41]

All of these diagnostic challenges reinforce the importance of considering trauma with most patient encounters and applying an organized approach to the information obtained. One such schema is to consider trauma when presented with mild (functional symptoms), moderate (meet DSM-5 criteria for trauma diagnoses), or severe (impacting multiple domains of functioning) (**Table 1**).

Treatment

Psychoeducation and caregiver guidance

The pediatric response to symptoms is to start with psychoeducation, or helping patients and families to understand why they see the symptoms, and first steps to

Table 1
Suggestions for pediatricians in recognizing and managing trauma symptoms based on risk level

Risk Level	Behavioral Functioning and Development	Parenting/Caregiving	Suggestions for Care Plan
Low	Typical	Competent caregiver consistently provides safe, stable, nurturing relationship; little-to-mild caregiver stress(ors)	Follow preventive health care plan; focus on strengthening protective factors and building resilience
Medium	Fairly typical to mildly atypical behavior or behavior changes	Competent-to-mild caregiver challenges; mild-to-medium caregiver stress(ors)	Suggestions for low-risk level, plus closer follow-up and monitoring with an increased attention to increasing regulation skills and supporting safe, stable, nurturing caregiving
High	Mild-to-moderate trauma-related symptoms	Mild-to-moderate caregiver challenges; moderate-to-high caregiver stress(ors)	Increase frequency and intensity for low and medium-risk interventions; add case management; connect with community partners; consider trauma-informed mental health services, including evidence-based treatments, if available
Severe	Moderate-to-severe trauma-related symptoms	Moderately to significant caregiver challenges; moderate-to-severe caregiver stress(ors)	Higher frequency and intensity of interventions earlier; increase office interventions and case management with referral to community services and trauma-focused evidence-based treatments, if available

Adapted from Heather C. Forkey, Jessica L. Griffin, Moira Szilagyi, Integrated care. (2021). In Childhood Trauma & Resilience: A Practical Guide, American Academy of Pediatrics. https://doi.org/10.1542/9781610025072-ch14.

respond. There are a number of online resources that have been developed to assist families when their child has experienced trauma. **Table 2** recommended resources; however, it is important to note that this is not an exhaustive list.

The next step is to provide simple strategies to help children recover. Pediatricians can start by promoting what we refer to as the “3 Rs,” which is a simple way to begin to promote a sense of safety for the child. The 3 Rs are reassurance, routines, and regulation.[42]

Reassurance refers to the idea that no matter what the traumatic experience has been, children need to know that they are safe and loved. Given the physiologic impact of trauma on the child’s brain and physiology, children who have experienced trauma often revert to not feeling safe in their environment—essentially having an overactive internal alarm system. Reassuring the child that they are safe is an essential

Table 2
Online resources for psychoeducation

Resource	Description of Resource	Audience	Link
National Child Traumatic Stress Network (NCTSN)	Psychoeducational materials and resources for children and families who experience trauma	Children, adolescents, young adults, caregivers, and child-serving professionals	NCTSN website
Sesame Street Workshop	Videos, worksheets, and other tools to promote mental health in young children	Children and caregivers	Sesame Workshop Link
Center on the Developing Child (Harvard)	Web site with videos and other resources providing psychoeducation on trauma, toxic stress, and resilience	Children, caregivers, and child-serving professionals	Center on the Developing Child
Dare to Share (Child Mind Institute)	Videos of celebrities and others talking about their own challenges and how they got help; Tip sheets for parents and youth	Children adolescents and caregivers	Dare to Share Link
Mental Health is Health (MTV Entertainment Studios)	Toolkit aiming to normalize conversation and provide resources on mental health	Adolescents and caregivers	Mental Health Is Health Link
Dougy Center	Psychoeducational resources for children and families on grief	Children and caregivers	Dougy Center
National Association for Children of Addiction (NACoA)	Psychoeducational resources addressing the impact of substance use on children and families	Children, adolescents, caregivers, and professionals	NACoA Link
Doing what matters in times of stress (WHO)	Toolkit for coping with stress and adversity available in multiple languages	Children, adolescents, and caregivers	WHO toolkit link
Help Kids Cope App	Helps parents to talk to their kids about natural disasters and know how best to support them	Caregivers, children, adolescents, and teachers	Help Kids Cope Link

element of a trauma-informed response. Caregivers can send messages of safety through their words (eg, you are safe, you are loved, and the grownups are doing everything they can to make sure you are safe), through their tone of voice and expression (using softer tones and welcoming body language), as well as physical touch when appropriate and with consent and caution (eg, hugs, snuggling, and rocking the child). Caregivers are advised not to overpromise, particularly with regard to things that are outside of their control or not plausible (eg, you'll never have to see that person again). It can be helpful to let parents/caregivers know that they may have to convey messages of reassurance frequently and consistently over time, even if they think the child already believes they are safe and loved.

Routines are a simple, yet highly effective, way to begin to send signals to the child's brain that they are safe. Setting structure in the form of routines can be calming for a child who has experienced the chaos of trauma. For caregivers who struggle with setting limits/routines for their child, letting them know that routines are calming can be a helpful message for parents who, out of their own guilt about what their child has experienced, have stopped setting limits. Asking a family about bedtime routines or morning or after school routines can be a good strategy to incorporate into your check-ins with families and can be a good place to start for a parent who is struggling with what to do. Routines do not need to be overly complicated. Rather a simple predictable pattern that a child can come to expect over time. For example, a bedtime routine could look like: an hour before bedtime the parent begins to lower lights, ends screen time and the child takes a bath, they read a book together, the parent sings them a familiar song, and they hug good night with lights out. It can also be helpful to post routines somewhere around the house (bedtime routine in the bathroom, afterschool routine on the refrigerator, and so forth).

The third R is *regulation* and consists of both calming the body's stress response through relaxation activities as well as identifying and expressing feelings more effectively. Relaxation activities could include things like belly breathing or deep breathing strategies, mindfulness activities, grounding strategies, progressive muscle relaxation, or other activities that may promote relaxation such as coloring, exercise, prayer, dance, listening to music, or other activity that involves the music or senses. There are a number of online tools and apps available to assist with relaxation as well (**Table 3**).

The second part of regulation involves helping children better identify how they are feeling by increasing their feelings' vocabulary and expressing their feelings more effectively. For children who lack the language to describe how they are feeling, they may be more apt to use maladaptive strategies. By increasing their feelings vocabulary, caregivers can help children have language to talk about uncomfortable experiences.

Other "prescriptions" could include prescribing "special time in," which is a strategy in which the caregiver picks the same time every day—whatever time works best for that family—and spending 10 minutes doing an activity with the child of the child's choosing (other than screen time where they are not interacting) where that parent is able to provide uninterrupted attuned attention to the child. Activities do not need to be elaborate and could include drawing together, playing a game, making a snack, playing with clay, having a dance party, shooting hoops, or other activity tailored to the child's age/developmental status. It can be helpful to have a list of activities they could do together. Critical to the success of this strategy is coaching the parent/caregiver to stick with this for at least 2 weeks, even if the child starts to "act out" toward the end of their special time with the caregiver—it does not mean they are doing it wrong, it likely means that child is getting what they need the most, one-on-one attuned connected time with their caregiver. We suggest 10 minutes because 10 minutes is manageable for most families, and we want parents to have some success with this. If 10 minutes feels overwhelming, start with 5 minutes.

Mental health referral

When initial supports are not effective and/or if the child is symptomatic, a referral to evidence-based treatment of child trauma may be warranted. There are many

Table 3
Relaxation apps for children and caregivers

Breathe, Think, Do with Sesame Street	Helps children 2–5 build resilience through problem-solving skills and teaches belly breathing	Preschool age children, teachers, and caregivers	Breathe, Think, Do Link
Calm App	Meditation/Mindfulness app to improve sleep, decrease stress and anxiety	All ages	https://www.calm.com
Headspace	Meditation/Mindfulness app to decrease stress and anxiety and improve sleep	All ages	https://www.headspace.com
Insight Timer App	Meditation/mindfulness app to improve sleep and mental health	All ages	https://insighttimer.com
Smiling Mind App	Offers mindfulness and meditation programs for all ages including age-specific programs	All ages	Smiling Mind Link
Super Stretch Yoga	Online tool and app that teaches importance of relaxation and breathing while incorporating body using yoga poses	Ages 4 y and above	https://adventuresofsuperstretch.com

evidence based treatments (EBTs) for child trauma that exist that can be applied in various settings (eg, home-based, outpatient, school-based, or residential/congregate care settings). The following are included as the most widely used or well-researched EBTs for childhood trauma, but the reader is informed that this is not an exhaustive list (**Table 4**). For further information about EBTs and the available research to support these, the reader is referred to Results First Clearinghouse Database, which is a clearinghouse of EBTs currently housed at Penn State University.

While an exhaustive discussion of all the types of evidence base trauma therapy is beyond the scope of this study, it can be very helpful to know what the critical elements of trauma-focused EBTs are.[54,55] Most communities in the United States have some access to some of these treatments, and beyond that, mental health providers may claim to provide trauma-informed or evidence-informed therapy. Elements to look for and questions to ask to determine if services offered are likely to be useful include

- Screening/assessment: When conducting trauma-informed treatment, it is recommended that clinicians use trauma screening and assessment tools to measure trauma exposure, trauma-related symptoms, strengths, and psychosocial functioning as well as to measure risk and determine that a trauma-focused treatment is warranted. Additionally, assessment can help to document treatment progress and determine when treatment is no longer indicated.
- Building a strong therapeutic relationship: Regardless of which treatment is being utilized, for treatment to be successful, it is critical that clinicians are able to effectively engage their clients and establish a strong therapeutic relationship with children and their caregivers.[56,57]
- Psychoeducation about normal responses to trauma: As described earlier, psychoeducation is an essential element of trauma-informed care. In treatment,

Table 4
Evidence-based treatments for trauma

Treatment	Web Site and National Roster of Trained Clinicians (When Available)	Age Range	Modality	Setting	Treatment Length
Trauma-focused cognitive-behavioral therapy[43,44]	www.tfcbt.org https://tfcbt.org/therapists	3–18 years	Individual, parent–child sessions, group format available	Outpatient, residential, inpatient, home-based, school-based	8–16 sessions; 16–25 for complex trauma
Child parent psychotherapy[45,46]	https://childparentpsychotherapy.com https://childtrauma.ucsf.edu/cpp-provider-roster	0–5 years	Parent–child dyad	Outpatient or home-based	52 wk, on average
Parent–child interaction therapy[47,48]	https://www.pcit.org https://www.pcit.org/find-a-provider.html	2–7 years	Parent–child dyad	Outpatient or home-based	12–20 sessions
Child and family traumatic stress intervention[49]	https://medicine.yale.edu/childstudy/services/community-and-schools-programs/yctsr/stress-intervention/	7–18 years	Individual and caregiver sessions	Outpatient	5–8 sessions
Attachment and biobehavioral catchup[50,51]	https://www.abcparenting.org/findaparentcoach/g	0–48 mo	Caregiver–child dyad	Home-visiting	10 sessions
Trauma affect regulation: Guide for education and therapy for adolescents[52,53]	https://www.atspro.org/targetcurricula	10–18 years	Individual sessions	Outpatient, juvenile justice, residential	10–12 sessions; occasionally fewer

clinicians provide general information about trauma and trauma-related symptoms and reactions, with the goal to normalize the child's symptoms and experiences. Psychoeducation can be a powerful tool to allow children and their caregivers to understand that it is not about what is wrong with them, but what has happened to them, and it provides hope that they can heal from their traumatic experiences.

- Parent/caregiver support/training, conjoint sessions: Clinicians need to be not just comfortable working with children, but engaging parents too. Caregiver engagement and support can help to decrease caregiver stress, strengthen the parent–child relationship, and help to reinforce the child learning and practicing coping and safety skills at home.
- Knowledge of child development: Without a solid knowledge base of what to expect from children at different developmental stages, a child's symptoms could be misinterpreted and the therapeutic approach and treatment misguided.
- Emotional expression and regulation skills: As an essential part of trauma-informed care, clinicians need to be adept at helping children identify their feelings, increase their feelings vocabulary, and express their feelings (including painful or uncomfortable ones) more effectively.
- Anxiety management and relaxation skills: In trauma-informed treatments, therapists provide relaxation and stress management skills in the form of relaxation training, helping children (and caregivers) turn down the stress response in the body through deep breathing, exercise, meditation or mindfulness, dance, or other activities.
- Cognitive processing or reframing: Children and adolescents who experienced trauma are prone to inaccurate or unhelpful thoughts (eg, "The world is a dangerous place," or "It's my fault I was abused," or "I am unlovable." Clinicians use a series of techniques in order to help children gently challenge these thoughts and come up with more accurate and helpful thoughts.
- Trauma narration and trauma processing: An important element of trauma-focused treatment is helping children be able to talk about what happened to them in a format and pace that is engaging and comfortable for them, while measuring their level of distress. Talking about trauma helps to promote desensitization to painful, frightening, or uncomfortable memories they have about the trauma and the resultant physiologic and emotional/behavioral response. Additionally, trauma narration helps to put it into a context for the child and assist them in making meaning out of what happened to them.
- Promoting safety: Lastly, but often most importantly, clinicians engage in promoting the child's physical safety through safety planning (usually with caregivers) to help youth identify safe relationships and situations and to prevent revictimization as well as promoting the child's psychological safety by helping youth and their caregivers identify potential trauma triggers or reminders and help to plan for what to do when they are reminded of their traumatic experiences.

Pediatric practices can facilitate referrals to EBTs in a number of ways. First, by providing psychoeducation about evidence-based treatment of trauma—an overview of what the treatment is, highlighting that they are all typically time-limited, and emphasizing hope for families—that healing is possible and that these are treatments that, just like medicines that are prescribed for their child, are shown to be more effective than treatment as usual or no treatment at all. Second, by explaining the importance of talking about trauma or exploring trauma in treatment. We have found it helpful to use the metaphor of cleaning out a wound. "Let's say you fall down and you get a scrape on your knee. What could you do about that scrape? You could ignore it and hope it gets better or you could take the time and clean out the wound. Not every wound gets infected, but for those that do, they can cause long-term problems and worsen. Talking about trauma is kind of like cleaning out that wound. By talking about it, we're trying to promote healing so that long-term problems don't happen...If I cleaned the wound too fast or too hard that could make it worse, so just like cleaning out a wound, you'll do it at a pace that's comfortable for you." Lastly, by checking in with the family to see whether they attended their appointment and discussing any barriers to accessing services. It can be helpful to explain that just like when their pediatrician suggests taking all of their medication (eg, an antibiotic), even if they are feeling better, that same principle applies. That in therapy, they may start to feel better as they learn coping skills, but it is important to finish the course of treatment in order to support long-term healing.

Medication

For the primary care physician, prescribing of medication to children with trauma symptoms can present a challenge. On the one hand, medication is never recommended as a first-line response for trauma. In contrast to the robust data supporting the use of evidence-based trauma therapy presented earlier, there are very limited data regarding the efficacy of medication for treating trauma in children, and data we do have suggest a higher risk of medication side effects in children exposed to trauma. Yet, the pediatric provider may feel pressure to prescribe in the face of behavioral challenges or crisis (especially for children involved with child welfare who have experienced repeated relational trauma, inconsistent health care, and poor access to safe stable caregivers). Alternatively, children can present to primary care already having been prescribed multiple medications to address trauma symptoms, including complex combinations of medications with significant side effect and risk profiles. That is why consideration of medication and the prescribing or deprescribing in the context of trauma should be done following use of the strategies laid out in the prior sections. This includes consideration of the patient's experience of trauma, situation and understanding of symptoms, the results of surveillance and screening, and careful consideration of the diagnosis and other conditions that could be confused with or comorbid with trauma. The reader is referred to the American Academy of Pediatrics and American Academy of Child and Adolescent Psychiatry combined clinical report on Children Exposed to Maltreatment: Assessment and the Role of Psychotropic Medication which reviews these issues, as well as current data and recommendations regarding medication in the population of children exposed to trauma.[58]

CLINICS CARE POINTS

- Begin TIC by preparing yourself and your team with training on trauma, its health consequences and strategies to mitigate these.
- Engage with families in ways that promote safety through language, body language, vocal tone, empathy, and curiosity.
- Screen for exposure and symptoms of trauma, particularly when combined with screening for conditions (ADHD, depression, anxiety) that have symptoms in common with trauma; this will guide diagnosis and management.
- The differential diagnosis of trauma can be challenging, but organizing the presentation into mild, moderate, or severe symptoms can help guide diagnosis.

- There are practical ways to explain trauma symptoms to children and families and help guide them to recognize and address those symptoms.
- Be knowledgeable about the various evidence-based treatment options available to address child trauma. Children may need referral to community resources, particularly evidence-based treatments.
- Providers can help to facilitate referrals to treatment by providing psychoeducation about why trauma treatment is beneficial and how it can be addressed through treatment.
- Medication has a very small role in the management of trauma and should be considered only after engaging psychosocial treatment and evidence-based therapy.

DISCLOSURE

Both Dr H. Forkey and Dr J. Griffin receive royalties from AAP Publications from sale of the book, Forkey H, Griffin, J, Szilagyi, M. *Childhood Trauma and Resilience: A Practical Guide.* Chicago, IL: American Academy of Pediatrics; 2021.

REFERENCES

1. Friedman M. PTSD History and Overview. In: U.S. Department of veterans affairs. PTSD: national center for PTSD web site. 2022. Available at: https://www.ptsd.va.gov/professional/treat/essentials/history_ptsd.asp. Accessed March 3, 2024.
2. Felitti VJ, Anda RF, Nordenberg D, et al. Relationship of childhood abuse and household dysfunction to many of the leading causes of death in adults. The Adverse Childhood Experiences (ACE) Study. Am J Prev Med 1998;14(4):245–58.
3. Anda RF, Felitti VJ, Bremner JD, et al. The enduring effects of abuse and related adverse experiences in childhood - A convergence of evidence from neurobiology and epidemiology. Eur Arch Psychiatr Clin Neurosci 2006;256(3):174–86.
4. De Bellis MD, Zisk A. The biological effects of childhood trauma. Child Adolesc Psychiatr Clin N Am 2014;23(2):185–222, vii.
5. Boyce WT, Levitt P, Martinez FD, et al. Genes, environments, and time: the biology of adversity and resilience. Pediatrics 2021;147(2):e20201651.
6. Danese A, McEwen BS. Adverse childhood experiences, allostasis, allostatic load, and age-related disease. Physiol Behav 2012;106(1):29–39.
7. Lupien SJ, McEwen BS, Gunnar MR, et al. Effects of stress throughout the lifespan on the brain, behaviour and cognition. Nat Rev Neurosci 2009;10(6):434–45.
8. McEwen BS, Gianaros PJ. Central role of the brain in stress and adaptation: links to socioeconomic status, health, and disease. Ann N Y Acad Sci 2010;1186:190–222.
9. Shonkoff JP, Boyce WT, McEwen BS. Neuroscience, molecular biology, and the childhood roots of health disparities: building a new framework for health promotion and disease prevention. JAMA 2009;301(21):2252–9.
10. Johnson SB, Riley AW, Granger DA, et al. The science of early life toxic stress for pediatric practice and advocacy. Pediatrics 2013;131(2):319–27.
11. Shonkoff JP, Garner AS, Committee on Psychosocial Aspects of Child and Family Health, et al. The lifelong effects of early childhood adversity and toxic stress. Pediatrics 2012;129(1):e232–46.
12. Gunnar M, Quevedo K. The neurobiology of stress and development. Annu Rev Psychol 2007;58:145–73.
13. Feldman R. What is resilience: an affiliative neuroscience approach. World Psychiatr 2020;19(2):132–50.

14. Taylor SE. Tend and befriend: biobehavioral bases of affiliation under stress. Curr Dir Psychol Sci 2006;15(6):273–7.
15. Bos PA. The endocrinology of human caregiving and its intergenerational transmission. Development and Psychopathology 2017;29(3):971–99.
16. Porges SW. Social engagement and attachment: a phylogenetic perspective. Ann N Y Acad Sci 2003;1008:31–47.
17. Bartz JA, Zaki J, Bolger N, et al. Social effects of oxytocin in humans: context and person matter. Trends Cognit Sci 2011;15(7):301–9.
18. Feldman R. Sensitive periods in human social development: new insights from research on oxytocin, synchrony, and high-risk parenting. Development and Psychopathology 2015;27(2):369–95.
19. Olff M, Frijling JL, Kubzansky LD, et al. The role of oxytocin in social bonding, stress regulation and mental health: an update on the moderating effects of context and interindividual differences. Psychoneuroendocrinology 2013;38(9):1883–94.
20. Shamay-Tsoory SG, Abu-Akel A. The social salience hypothesis of oxytocin. Biol Psychiatr 2016;79(3):194–202.
21. Garner A, Yogman M, Committee on Psychosocial Aspects of Child And Family Health, Section on Developmental And Behavioral Pediatrics, Council on Early Childhood. Preventing childhood toxic stress: partnering with families and communities to promote relational health. Pediatrics 2021;148(2). e2021052582.
22. National Child Traumatic Stress Network. Creating trauma informed systems. 2016. Available at: https://www.nctsn.org/trauma-informed-care/creating-trauma-informed-systems. Accessed March 23, 2024.
23. Duffee J, Szilagyi M, Forkey H, et al, Council on Community Pediatrics, Council on Foster Care, Adoption, and Kinship Care, Council on Child Abuse and Neglect, Committee on Psychosocial Aspects of Child And Family Health. Trauma-informed care in child health systems. Pediatrics 2021;148(2). e2021052579.
24. Substance Abuse and Mental Health Services Administration. SAMHSA's Concept of Trauma and Guidance for a Trauma-Informed Approach. 2022. Available at: https://www.samhsa.gov/resource/dbhis/samhsas-concept-trauma-guidance-trauma-informed-approach. Accessed February 23, 2024.
25. Purewal SKB, Monica W, Gutiérrez L, et al. Screening for adverse childhood experiences (ACEs) in an integrated pediatric care model. Zero Three 2016;36(3):10–7.
26. Baldwin JR, Caspi A, Meehan AJ, et al. Population vs individual prediction of poor health from results of adverse childhood experiences screening. Pediatrics 2021; 175(4):385–93.
27. Anda RF, Porter LE, Brown DW. Inside the adverse childhood experience score: strengths, limitations, and misapplications. Am J Prev Med 2020;59(2):293–5.
28. Forkey H, Szilagyi M, Kelly ET, Council on Community Pediatrics, Council on Foster Care, Adoption, and Kinship Care, Council on Child Abuse and Neglect, Committee on Psychosocial Aspects of Child and Family Health, et al. Trauma-informed care. Pediatrics 2021;148(2). e2021052580.
29. Porges SW. neuroception: a subconscious system for detecting threats and safety. Zero Three 2004;24:19–24.
30. Hughes DA, Baylin J. The neurobiology of attachment-focused therapy: enhancing connection and trust in the treatment of children and adolescents. New York: W.W. Norton & Company; 2016.
31. Sheldrick RC, Perrin EC. Evidence-based milestones for surveillance of cognitive, language, and motor development. Academic Pediatrics 2013;13(6):577–86.

32. Dubowitz H, Feigelman S, Lane W, et al. Pediatric primary care to help prevent child maltreatment: the Safe Environment for Every Kid (SEEK) model. Pediatrics 2009;123(3):858–64.
33. Keeshin B, Byrne K, Thorn B, et al. Screening for trauma in pediatric primary care. Curr Psychiatr Rep 2020;22(11):60.
34. Sachser C, Berliner L, Risch E, et al. The Child and Adolescent Trauma Screen 2 (CATS-2) - validation of an instrument to measure DSM-5 and ICD-11 PTSD and complex PTSD in children and adolescents. Eur J Psychotraumatol 2022;13(2): 2105580.
35. Lang JM, Connell CM. Development and validation of a brief trauma screening measure for children: The Child Trauma Screen. Psychological Trauma: Theory, Research. Practice and Policy 2017;9(3):390–8.
36. Rolon-Arroyo B, Oosterhoff B, Layne CM, et al. The UCLA PTSD Reaction Index for DSM-5 brief form: a screening tool for trauma-exposed youths. J Am Acad Child Adolesc Psychiatry 2020;59(3):434–43.
37. Foa EB, Asnaani A, Zang Y, et al. Psychometrics of the Child PTSD Symptom Scale for DSM-5 for Trauma-Exposed Children and Adolescents. J Clin Child Adolesc Psychol 2018;47(1):38–46.
38. Foa EB, Johnson KM, Feeny NC, et al. The Child PTSD Symptom Scale: a preliminary examination of its psychometric properties. J Clin Child Psychol 2001;30(3): 376–84.
39. Teicher MHSJ, Samson JA. Childhood maltreatment and psychopathology: A case for ecophenotypic variants as clinically and neurobiologically distinct subtypes. Am J Psychiatr 2013;170(10):1114–33.
40. Ford JD. Complex PTSD: research directions for nosology/assessment, treatment, and public health. Eur J Psychotraumatol 2015;6:27584.
41. Spinazzola J, van der Kolk B, Ford JD. Developmental trauma disorder: A legacy of attachment trauma in victimized children. J Trauma Stress 2021;34(4):711–20.
42. Forkey H, Griffin J, Szilagyi M. Childhood trauma and resilience: a practical guide. Chicago, IL: American Academy of Pediatrics; 2021.
43. Cohen JA, Deblinger E, Mannarino AP, et al. A multisite, randomized controlled trial for children with sexual abuse-related PTSD symptoms. J Am Acad Child Adolesc Psychiatry 2004;43(4):393–402.
44. Cohen JA, Mannarino AP, Deblinger E. Treating trauma and traumatic grief in children and adolescents. 2nd edition. New York, NY, US: Guilford Press; 2017.
45. Lieberman AF, Ghosh Ippen C, Van Horn P. Child-Parent Psychotherapy: *6-month follow-up of a randomized controlled trial.* J Am Acad Child Adolesc Psychiatry 2006;45(8):913–8.
46. Dickstein S. Alicia F. Lieberman, Chandra Ghosh Ippen, and Patricia Van Horn, Don't hit my mommy! A manual for child-parent psychotherapy with young children exposed to violence and other trauma (2nd edition). Washington, DC: Zero to Three; 2015.
47. Eyberg SM, Boggs SR, Algina J. Parent-child interaction therapy: A psychosocial model for the treatment of young children with conduct problem behavior and their families. Psychopharmacol Bull 1995;31(1):83–91.
48. Funderburk BW, Eyberg S. Parent–child interaction therapy. In: History of psychotherapy: continuity and change. 2nd edition. Washington, DC, US: American Psychological Association; 2011. p. 415–20.
49. Berkowitz SJ, Stover CS, Marans SR. The Child and Family Traumatic Stress Intervention: secondary prevention for youth at risk of developing PTSD. J Child Psychol Psychiatry Allied Discip 2011;52(6):676–85.

50. Dozier M, Bernard K, Roben CKP. Attachment and biobehavioral catch-up. In: Steele HaS M, editor. Handbook of attachment-based interventions. New York , NY: The Guilford Press; 2018. p. 27–49.
51. Dozier M, Peloso E, Lindhiem O, et al. Developing evidence-based interventions for foster children: an example of a randomized clinical trial with infants and toddlers. J Soc Issues 2006;62(4):767–85.
52. Ford J. Trauma affect regulation: Guide for education and therapy. In: Ford J, Curtois C, editors. Treating complex traumatic stress disorders in adults: scientific foundations and therapeutic models. 2nd edition. New York, NY: The Guilford Press; 2020. p. 390–412.
53. Ford JD, Karen LS, Hawke JM, et al. Randomized trial comparison of emotion regulation and relational psychotherapies for ptsd with girls involved in delinquency. J Clin Child Adolesc Psychol 2012;41(1):27–37.
54. Strand VC, Hansen S, Courtney DM. Common elements across evidence-based trauma treatment: discovery and implications. Adv Soc Work 2013;14:334–54.
55. Kooij LH, van der Pol TM, Daams JG, et al. Common elements of evidence-based trauma therapy for children and adolescents. Eur J Psychotraumatol 2022;13(1): 2079845.
56. Ardito RB, Rabellino D. Therapeutic alliance and outcome of psychotherapy: historical excursus, measurements, and prospects for research. Front Psychol 2011;2:270.
57. Ormhaug SM, Jensen TK, Wentzel-Larsen T, et al. The therapeutic alliance in treatment of traumatized youths: relation to outcome in a randomized clinical trial. J Consult Clin Psychol 2014;82(1):52–64.
58. Keeshin B, Forkey HC, Fouras G, et al, American Academy Of Pediatrics, Council On Child Abuse And Neglect, Council On Foster Care, Adoption, And Kinship Care, American Academy Of Child And Adolescent Psychiatry, Committee On Child Maltreatment And Violence, Committee On Adoption And Foster Care. Children exposed to maltreatment: assessment and the role of psychotropic medication. Pediatrics 2020;145(2):e20193751. https://doi.org/10.1542/peds.2019-3751.

Evidence-Based Youth Suicide Prevention and Intervention in Pediatric Primary Care Settings

Donna A. Ruch, PhD[a,b,*], Jennifer L. Hughes, PhD, MPH[c,d], Jeffrey A. Bridge, PhD[a,b,c,d], Cynthia A. Fontanella, PhD[a,d]

KEYWORDS

- Pediatric primary care • Youth suicide • Evidence-based practice

KEY POINTS

- Youth suicide is a major public health concern.
- Primary care practices are increasingly faced with addressing youth mental health concerns.
- Evidence-based screening, assessment, and management strategies can aid pediatric primary care providers in youth suicide prevention efforts.
- Enhanced residency and continuing medical education training opportunities can better equip pediatric primary care providers to manage suicide risk.
- Future research is needed to evaluate the clinical pathway effectiveness in primary care settings.

INTRODUCTION

Suicide is a leading cause of death among youth aged 10 to 19 years in the United States and in 2022 accounted for 23% of all deaths in this age group.[1] Following a steady decline since 1999, suicide rates in this age group increased 27% between 2011 and 2022 (from 4.9 to 6.3 per 100,000).[2] Suicidal ideation, defined as thoughts

[a] Center for Suicide Prevention and Research, The Abigail Wexner Research Institute at Nationwide Children's Hospital, 444 Butterfly Gardens Drive, Columbus, OH 43205, USA; [b] Department of Pediatrics, The Ohio State University College of Medicine, 1645 Neil Avenue, Columbus, OH 43210, USA; [c] Big Lots Behavioral Health Services and Division of Child and Family Psychiatry, Nationwide Children's Hospital, 444 Butterfly Gardens Drive, Columbus, OH 43205, USA; [d] Department of Psychiatry and Behavioral Health, The Ohio State University College of Medicine, 1645 Neil Avenue, Columbus, OH 43210, USA

* Corresponding author. Center for Suicide Prevention and Research, The Abigail Wexner Research Institute at Nationwide Children's Hospital, 444 Butterfly Gardens Drive, Columbus, OH 43205.

E-mail address: donna.ruch@Nationwidechildrens.org

Pediatr Clin N Am 71 (2024) 1119–1140
https://doi.org/10.1016/j.pcl.2024.07.017 pediatric.theclinics.com

of ending one's life, and suicide attempts, a non-fatal self-injurious behavior with stated or inferred intent to die, have also increased substantially in youth, and are strong predictors of future suicide.[3] According to the 2021 Youth Risk Behavior Survey of US high school students, 22% of youth indicated they seriously considered suicide, and 10% of youth reported they attempted suicide at least once in the prior 12 month.[4]

Primary care practices are a major point of contact for health care services and youth who may be at risk for suicide, and in some cases the de facto mental health care setting.[5] A 2019 survey by the American Academy of Pediatrics (AAP) found over 90% of pediatricians had a patient screen positive or disclose suicide ideation, and 81% reported having a patient who attempted or died by suicide.[6] Research further shows approximately 80% of suicide decedents are seen by primary care providers in the year prior to death, while only 20% have contact with a mental health professional.[7,8] This is particularly concerning for rural and underserved communities where economic, geographic, or cultural barriers may limit access to mental health services.[9,10] Also, many youth would prefer to see their primary care provider concerning emotional problems, as there is less stigma and more accessibility.

Evidence highlights the importance of identifying youth at risk for suicide in pediatric primary care and suggests this is an essential setting for improving youth mental and behavioral health. The AAP also recommends that primary care providers not only screen and assess for suicide risk, but also become educated on how to manage certain mental health conditions and more effectively link patients to necessary specialized care and follow-up services.[11] Although research has advanced many effective strategies to prevent youth suicide, continued efforts are needed to address this pressing public health problem. This article will discuss the current epidemiology of youth suicide in the United States and describe research and evidence-based best strategies for suicide prevention in pediatric primary care including suicide risk screening, assessment, intervention, follow-up monitoring, and innovative practices.

Epidemiology of Youth Suicide

Age/Sex

Youth suicide and suicidal behavior are associated with risk factors across multiple domains including individual (eg, psychopathology, prior suicidal behavior), family (eg, familial suicide, family discord, child maltreatment), and social (eg, school/peer-related problems, media effects)[12] (**Box 1**). Developmental and demographic factors also influence rates of youth suicide. Between 2001 and 2021, youth suicide rates in males were 3 times higher than females and represented 77% of all suicide deaths in 10- to 19-year-olds[2] (**Fig. 1**). However, recent data reveal a narrowing gap between male and female youth suicide.[2,13] Regarding age, suicide rates among youth aged 10 to 14 years increased 59% between 2012 and 2022 (from 1.4 to 2.4 per 100,000), compared to a 20% increase in youth aged 15 to 19 years (from 8.3 to 10.0 per 100,000)[2]; females aged 10 to 14 years showed the sharpest increase, with suicide rates more than doubling during this timeframe (from 0.8 to 1.9 per 100,000).[2]

Race/ethnicity

American Indian/Alaska Native (AI/AN) youth experience the highest rates of suicide in the United States[2] (**Fig. 2**). From 2018 to 2022, the suicide rate among AI/AN youth aged 10 to 19 years in the United States (25.8 per 100,000) was 3 times the rate for white youth (7.8 per 100,000), and over 4 times higher than rates for black, Asian/

Box 1
Risk factors for youth suicide

Individual
- Mental Health Concerns
- Substance Abuse
- Previous Suicidal Behavior
- Interpersonal Loss/trauma
- Physical and sexual abuse
- Medical illness
- Impulsivity/Aggression
- Sexual minority/gender identity

Family/Peer
- Conflicting Family/Peer Relationships
- Childhood Trauma
- Family Violence
- Family History of Mental Health Disorders
- Family History of Suicide
- Family Stress

Community
- Lack of supportive relationships
- Barriers to health care services
- Lethal means access
- Unsafe media portrayals of suicide

Pacific Islander, and Hispanic youth.[2] Differences by race/ethnicity have also been identified in suicide rates among younger children. Bridge and colleagues,[14] found the suicide rate in children younger than 13 years to be roughly 2 times higher for black children compared with white children.

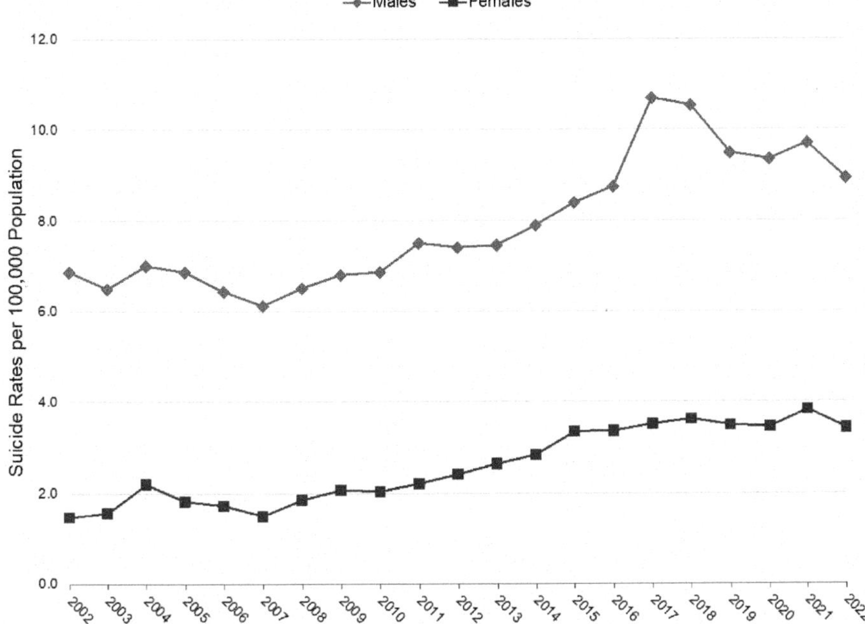

Fig. 1. US Youth suicide rates: Ages 10 to 19 years, 2002 to 2022.

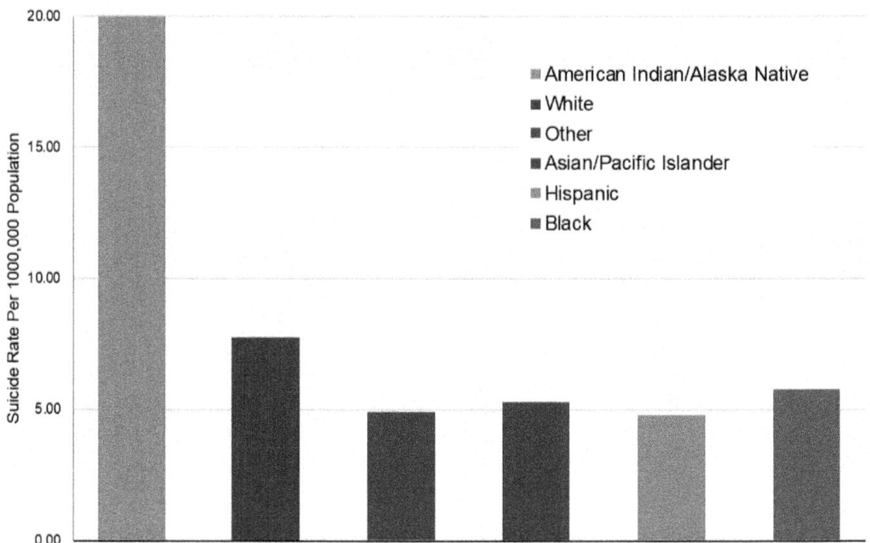

Fig. 2. US Youth suicide rates by race/ethnicity: Ages 10 to 19 years, 2018 to 2022.

Sexual and gender minority youth

Sexual and gender minority youth are also at greater risk for suicide than their peers. Raifman and colleagues,[15] evaluated youth sexual orientation and suicide attempts among US high school students from 2009 to 2017 and found students identifying as sexual minorities were more than 3 times as likely to attempt suicide compared to heterosexual students. An additional study showed bisexual youth were associated with significantly more suicide risk factors (depression, trauma, victimization) and less protective factors (parent-family connectedness, positive affect), along with elevated rates of both ideation and attempts compared to heterosexual and other sexual minority youth.[16]

Psychopathology

Research consistently shows a significant association between youth suicide and mental health issues,[17,18] which includes previous suicide attempts, the most robust clinical predictor of a future suicide attempt.[14,19] Depression is strongly linked to youth suicidal thoughts and behaviors (Nock and colleagues, 2013), and a national survey shows 19.5% of youth aged 12 to 17 years experienced a past year major depressive episode in 2022.[20] Comorbidity of mental health issues and substance abuse disorders are also shown to significantly increase the risk for youth suicide and suicidal behavior.[21]

Family factors

Multiple family-related factors have been linked to youth suicide. A study examining the familial transmission of suicidal behavior showed children of parents with a history of mood disorders and suicide attempts had a 5-fold increased odds of suicide attempt.[22] A study of children aged 9 to 10 years found family conflict and low parental monitoring were significantly associated with suicidal ideation even after controlling for demographic and psychosocial variables.[23] Studies further indicate increased risk for suicide due to parental loss from death, divorce, or abandonment.[24] Child maltreatment is also a significant risk for youth suicide, suicide attempts, and suicidal ideation[12,25,26]; a meta-analysis examining specific types of child maltreatment found sexual abuse to be the most significant predictor of future suicidal behavior (Angelakis and colleagues, 2020; Gomez and colleagues, 2017).[25,26]

Peer relations

Using data from 48 countries, a global study found bullying victimization was associated with a 3-fold increased odds of suicide attempt among youth aged 12 to 15 years.[27] An additional study assessed bullying and suicidal ideation in patients aged 12 to 17 years presenting to an emergency department with mental health issues.[28] Slightly more than 75% of youth indicated they experienced bullying at some point during their lives. Findings further revealed that victims of bullying were 9 times more likely to report suicidal ideation than youth with no history of bullying.[28] Previous research also suggests suicidal behaviors are influenced by affiliation with peers who have engaged in suicidal behaviors,[29] however positive peer influence is shown to be effective in school-based suicide prevention programs.[30,31]

Media/social media effects

A systematic review investigating social media/internet use and suicide attempts in youth aged 11 to 18 years found more frequent social media/internet use was associated with increased odds (1.03–5.10) for suicide attempt.[32] In an additional review, up to 25% of studies suggested positive aspects of social/media internet use, revealing youth with a history of suicidal behavior used the internet as a form of support and sense of community to seek help and connect with others.[33] Another concern is media contagion effects, referring to the media's direct and indirect influence on youth suicidal behavior. Recent studies indicate that sensational reports of celebrity suicide deaths that disregard reporting guidelines[34] and irresponsible fictional accounts of suicide such as those found in 13 Reasons Why Season 1[35] may increase the rate of suicides in the population.

Evidence-Based Strategies for Suicide Prevention in Pediatric Primary Care

Suicide risk screening

Early identification of suicide risk in youth is a critical step in suicide prevention, yet many youths often go undetected. To address this issue, many health care settings have implemented routine suicide risk screening. The AAP recommends that all pediatric patients be screened for depression annually, and to also inquire about factors shown to be associated with elevated suicide risk.[11] In the Blueprint for Youth Suicide Prevention, the AAP and the American Foundation for Suicide Prevention (AFSP), in collaboration with the National Institute of Mental Health (NIMH), more specifically call for universal suicide risk screening in youth ages 12 years and older in primary care and other clinical settings. The AAP further recommends youth aged 8 to 11 years be screened when clinically indicated, such as presenting with mental health concerns, or if there is a known history of suicidal thoughts and behaviors. For younger youth, guidelines suggest screening if there are warning signs of suicide risk or parental reports of youth suicidal thoughts and behaviors.

Suicide is closely linked with depression, and screening for depression is often the gateway to suicide prevention in primary care settings. A commonly used evidence-based depression screening instrument is the Patient Health Questionnaire PHQ-9.[36,37] While depression screening is important, research shows screening for depression alone is not adequate to detect suicide risk, and that not all youth at risk for suicide have depression symptoms.[16,38] In a study among medical inpatients aged 10 to 21 years, 39.5% of participants who screened positive for suicide risk did not screen positive for depression using the Patient Health Questionnaire-Adolescent Version (PHQ-A), and 56% did not report thoughts of self-harm or "being better off dead" on item 9 of the

PHQ-A.[16] An additional study found that suicide specific screening identified an additional 8.3% of patients aged 12 to 20 years at risk for suicide compared to depression screening alone.[38]

Evidence suggests screening for both depression and suicide risk can significantly detect more individuals with elevated risk for engaging in suicidal behavior.[16] To facilitate this process, the AAP recommends brief and easy to administer youth suicide screening tools to effectively guide clinicians in the assessment of suicide risk in pediatric care. One such evidence-based screening tool developed specifically for youth in medical settings is the Ask Suicide-Screening Questions (ASQ).[39,40] The ASQ is comprised of 4 initial questions that assess suicide ideation and suicidal behavior to identify patients who may need further risk assessment. A "yes" response or nonresponse to any of these questions results in a positive screening result for suicide risk, and prompts a fifth question to assess acuity.[40] Studies show the ASQ has high sensitivity, specificity, and negative predictive validity, and that it can detect patients at risk for suicide that depression screening alone fails to identify.[40–42] Additional risk screening tools shown to be effective in youth populations include the Suicidal Ideation Questionnaire,[43] Youth Suicide Ideation Screen,[44] and the Concise Health Risk Tracking Self-Report.[45]

Suicide assessment

Following a positive screen, assessment is a comprehensive evaluation, typically conducted by a medical provider or mental health clinician, to obtain more specific information about risk and protective factors, including diagnostic and psychosocial considerations, to guide next steps.[46,47] Commonly used assessment tools in pediatric primary care include the ASQ-Brief Suicide Safety Assessment (BSSA), Columbia Suicide Severity Rating Scale (C-SSRS), and the Suicide Assessment 5-Step Evaluation and Triage (SAFE-T).[47]

The BSSA was developed as a brief (15 minute) tool for clinicians/providers to aid in classification of risk to guide determining the next steps in care. The BSSA is part of the NIMH ASQ Suicide Risk Screening Toolkit (http://www.nimh.nih.gov/ASQ) and includes the following steps: (1) *Praise patient*, by expressing appreciation for disclosing their suicidal thoughts and/or behaviors; (2) *Assess the patient*, including asking about frequency of suicidal thoughts, presence of suicide plan, past self-injurious and/or suicidal behavior, psychiatric symptoms, and social support and stressors; (3) *Interview patient and parent/guardian together*, to elicit parent's perspectives on any assessed aspects discussed earlier as well as any family/friend history of suicide attempt, parental comfort with keeping child safe at home, and potentially dangerous items in home; (4) *Make a safety plan with the patient*, which includes coping strategies, means restriction guidance, and asking about self-efficacy related to keeping safe; (5) *Determine disposition*, such as whether patient is at imminent risk requiring emergency psychiatric evaluation, whether further evaluation is necessary via urgent 72 hour mental health referral, or whether a non-urgent mental health referral is needed; and (6) *Provide resources to all patients*, such as 988 and/or other local crisis resources. There are no psychometric validation studies of the BSSA at this time, though providers have reported this approach is acceptable.[47–49]

The C-SSRS (http://www.cssrs.columbia.edu/) is a tool to aid providers/clinicians in assessing more detailed suicide risk elements, including suicidal ideation, the intensity of suicidal ideation (including frequency, duration, controllability, deterrents, and reasons for ideation), suicidal behaviors and preparation (including actual attempts, interrupted attempts, aborted attempts, and preparatory acts or behaviors), and lethality (including actual and potential). The C-SSRS Risk Assessment version also includes an initial page with a checklist of risk and protective factors (eg, past week suicidal and self-injurious behavior, activating events, treatment history). The C-SSRS has demonstrated convergent validity with established suicidal ideation and behavior scales and strong divergent validity with depression scales.[47]

The SAFE-T, developed from the American Psychiatric Association Practice Guidelines for the Assessment and Treatment of Patients with Suicidal Behaviors, includes a 5-step process: (1) identify risk factors; (2) identify protective factors; (3) conduct suicide inquiry, including suicidal thoughts, plans, behavior, and intent; (4) determine risk level/intervention; and (5) document. The SAFE-T has frequently been used in primary care training and practice, though was not included as a suggested suicide risk assessment tool by the American Academy of Child and Adolescent Psychiatry (AACAP) Pathways in Clinical Care (PaCC) Workgroup.[50]

Suicide risk assessment should use systematic tools, include interviews with the child patient and parent/guardian, and result in informed clinical judgment regarding an immediate and longer-term disposition plan. Given their inclusion in the PaCC Workgroup recommendations for clinical pathways to address suicide risk in pediatric hospitals, the BSSA or C-SSRS are recommended as follow-up to a positive ASQ screen in pediatric primary care.[50] It is vital for providers to consider the cultural, societal, institutional, neighborhood, and family context in interpreting assessment findings.[51] These contextual factors have potentially differential implications for diagnosis and treatment in youth of color and minoritized youth who may experience poorer or delayed access to care.[47,51]

Pediatric providers should discuss with patients what to expect with regard to parent/guardian involvement during the assessment process. The Blueprint for Youth Suicide Prevention emphasizes having confidential, one-on-one time between the clinician and patient during clinic visit to discuss mental health and suicide risk. This conversation should include reviewing confidentiality and any limits and specific planning for how suicide risk information will be disclosed to the parent (ie, give patient a choice as to whether they want to be present or not when safety concerns are discussed with parent). The provider may meet with the parent individually after the suicide risk disclosure to answer questions about the child's safety and to more thoroughly discuss any action steps related to lethal means restriction or care planning.

Brief suicide interventions

Youth suicide screening and assessment practices must include management strategies to address both immediate and longer-term safety needs. Given the difficulties in accessing specialty mental health care and the high treatment dropout rates, pediatric primary care is the setting in which many youth with recent suicidal crises are likely to present. Families report seeing their pediatric primary care providers as someone who can help during times of suicidal crisis.[52] This underscores the need for screening, assessment and brief interventions to address safety, lethal means restriction counseling, and motivation/problem-solving to support mental health care linkage in this setting.

Brief youth suicide prevention interventions have been most robustly tested in emergency department (ED) settings, despite holding strong potential for effectiveness and current use across a wide variety of care settings, through implementation by a wide variety of care providers. Asarnow and colleagues[53] demonstrated that a brief family-based ED intervention, the Family Intervention for Suicide Prevention (FISP), could effectively link youth and parents to care and this intervention was effectively delivered in the ED setting in 80.9% of patients.[54] This approach has recently been adapted for use with pediatricians and is being piloted with pediatricians across Texas.

A recent meta-analysis of studies comparing safety-planning type interventions to control conditions included 6 studies in adult samples reporting outcomes on at least one of the following: suicidal behavior, suicide attempts, death by suicide, or suicidal ideation.[55] The meta-analysis found risk of suicidal behavior was significantly reduced by 43% [number needed to treat = 16] in the intervention conditions. In the 3 studies that included outcomes on suicidal ideation, there was no significant effect of safety planning. Safety plans appear to support behavior change for suicide prevention but may not impact levels of cognitive distress related to suicidal ideation.[56] Safety plans do increase self-efficacy and coping.[57,58] Studies have shown that clinicians report safety plans help get patients linked to care.[59] Of note, in this meta-analysis: (1) safety planning was operationalized as the safety plan containing, as a minimum, personalized coping strategies and sources of support; (2) all studies included development of the safety plan collaboratively with the clinician; (3) the safety plan was provided in person, on paper, or sent by mail. In 4 of the studies, the safety plan also included developing a list of personal warning signs of a suicidal crisis.[55] 2 commonly used approaches to safety planning with suicidal youth include the Safety Planning Intervention (SPI) and the FISP (also known as SAFETY-Acute). **Table 1** describes the core components of these 2 approaches, as well as their similarities and differences.

SPI is a brief intervention that has been included as a best practice strategy by the Suicide Prevention Resource Center (SPRC)/AFSP.[60,61] In SPI, the safety plan is a hierarchically arranged, written list of coping strategies and sources of support that the adolescent can use in a suicidal "crisis" or to avert such a crisis.[61] The safety plan is the product of a collaborative process between the provider and the patient, and to an appropriate extent, the parents. SPI was initially developed as part of the cognitive-behavioral therapy for suicide prevention (CBT-SP) intervention in the NIMH-funded Treatment of Adolescent Suicide Attempters study.[60,62] The current standalone SPI[63] intervention combines SPI and telephone follow-up, with the goal of contacting patients at least 2 times to monitor suicide risk, review and revise the SPI, and support treatment engagement. Patients who received the intervention were less likely to engage in suicidal behavior (3.03%) versus usual care (5.29%) during 6 months of follow-up.[63] An ongoing study is testing SPI with structured follow-up (SPI+) with adolescents.[64]

FISP, also included as an evidence-based intervention by SPRC/AFSP, is an enhanced mental health intervention involving a family-based CBT session in the ED designed to increase motivation for follow-up treatment, support, coping, and safety.[53] FISP is also the first session in an evidence-based outpatient intervention for youth with a recent suicide attempt, SAFETY.[65–68] FISP is a second-generation adaptation of the Specialized Emergency Room Intervention for Suicidal Adolescent Females,[69] which was designed with the primary goal of increasing linkage to outpatient mental health services. Primary targets of FISP are: (1) to directly address short-term risk of repeated suicidal behavior through enhancing motivation to seek follow-up treatment, strengthening youth and family coping skills, and educating the family about restricting access to potentially lethal means; (2) to educate about the importance of linking to follow-up care. FISP was tested in a randomized controlled trial in which suicidal youths at 2 EDs (N = 181; aged 10–18) were individually randomized to (1) Usual ED Care enhanced by provider education (UC); or (2) FISP, supplemented by care linkage telephone contacts after discharge. Intervention patients were significantly more likely to attend outpatient treatment compared to UC patients (92.1% vs 76.2%, $P = .004$).[53] The intervention group also had a significantly higher rate of psychotherapy, combined psychotherapy/medication, and

Table 1
Core components and comparisons of 2 safety planning approaches

Core Component	SPI	FISP	Similarities/Differences
Written Safety Plan Document	Hierarchically arranged list of coping strategies. Participant and parent/caregiver (if applicable) receive copy of written safety plan	Collaboratively developed safety plan, including behavioral and cognitive coping strategies. Provides youth with concrete tools, including a "safety plan card" to support safety after discharge	In FISP, tied to youth's individualized risk using "emotional thermometer" where youth identify feelings, triggers/thoughts/behaviors
Individualized to Participant Risk	Identify personalized warning signs for an impending suicide crisis	Provide family and youth with effective way to conceptualize the hierarchy of suicide-related situations using an "emotional thermometer"	In FISP, distress tolerance skills taught in this process and family is included.
Internal Coping Strategies	Determine internal coping strategies that distract from suicidal thoughts and urges	Identify coping strategies, such as distraction/self-soothing techniques, helpful thoughts, and ideas for a hope kit	In FISP, hope kit developed
Engaging Support System	Identify family and friends to distract from suicidal thoughts and urges; social places for interaction; individuals who can provide support during suicidal crisis	Develop a list of supportive individuals	SPI includes discussion of friends/family and place that can provide distraction, in addition to individuals who can provide support
Identification of Mental Health Supports	Develop a list mental health of professionals and urgent care services to contact during a suicidal crisis	Provide psychoeducation regarding the importance of youths receiving outpatient mental health treatment	SPI includes section on safety plan with specific services; FISP includes psychoeducation with youth and parents regarding importance of follow-up care

(*continued on next page*)

Table 1
(*continued*)

Core Component	SPI	FISP	Similarities/Differences
Focus on Protective Factors	Meet any discussion of protective factors with enthusiasm and interest to underscore existing coping and supports	Highlight and reinforce strengths and protective factors in youth and family through discussion of positive attributes and interactions to enhance family support and communication	FISP specifically includes activity "positives" to elicit youth and family strengths
Lethal Means Restriction Counseling	Lethal means restriction counseling for making the environment safe	Lethal means restriction counseling for making the environment safe	Similar in both SPI and FISP; conducted separately with parent/caregiver and youth
Follow-up Phone Calls	Contacts made within 72 h after discharge. 3 components: (1) brief risk assessment/mood check; (2) review and revision of SPI, if needed; and (3) facilitation of treatment engagement. Weekly follow-up phone calls concluding after 2 calls if patient attended at least one outpatient behavioral health appointment or no longer wished to be contacted.	Telephone contacts to enhance linkage to outpatient mental health care. First call made within the first 48 h after ED or hospital discharge with additional contacts as needed (usually at 1, 2, and 4 wk after discharge). Structured Phone calls, focused on enhancing motivation for seeking treatment, and providing referrals as needed to youths and families.	SPI phone calls include brief assessment of risk and mood, as well as review of safety plan, and linking to care. FISP phone calls only focus on linking to care.

more psychotherapy visits, but no significant effects on suicidality or other clinical/functioning outcomes (exploratory analyses).[53]

Lethal means restriction, or efforts to limit a person's access to methods which may be used to attempt suicide, have demonstrated efficacy lowering suicide rates.[70] Lethal means restriction counseling provided to parents of youth in the ED resulted in parents being 4 times more likely to restrict their child's access.[71] In a survey of pediatric primary care providers, only 19.4% reported consistently screening for firearms or providing lethal means restriction counseling.[72]

The American Board of Pediatrics and the AAP have called for increased training of pediatricians in managing patients with behavioral and mental health concerns, with the AAP specifically developing an educational resource for youth suicide prevention: "Suicide: Blueprint for Youth Suicide Prevention."[73] Given the impact on preventing suicidal behavior,[55] safety planning should continue to be identified as best practice for the prevention of suicidal behavior in individuals at risk of suicide, and should be strongly recommended in clinical practice and guidelines for suicide prevention. The AAP, SPRC, and the National Institute for Health and Care Excellence recommend safety planning for youth presenting with elevated suicide risk.

While the primary purpose of a safety plan is for the individual, in collaboration with the clinician, to identify personalized coping strategies to be used when experiencing suicidal thoughts or urges, a safety plan also includes individual suicide warning signs, resources for contacting social and professional support, including crisis lines and emergency services, and a focus on reducing access to lethal means. Motivational interviewing strategies, which are often used to address health behavior change in pediatric primary care, may enhance adherence to youth safety plan use and parents' motivation to encourage safety plan use.[57,58] Pediatric providers may consider using "Lock and Protect," a user-friendly web-based tool for parents to support lethal means counseling efforts with parents/caregivers.[74] This decisional aid uses behavioral economics approaches, such as "nudges" to guide parents through important considerations for home safety, such as who can help them take steps to lock up potentially dangerous means, which rooms in the house to consider, what they might need to secure items (such as a lockbox), and how to initiate crisis services if needed. Parents are provided with a personalized storage plan with action steps.[74] This tool is currently available at https://ucla.chsprc.com/.

Follow-up Care and Monitoring

Ensuring that youth at risk for suicide receive timely, seamless, uninterrupted follow-up care as they transition from one health setting to another has the potential to save lives and reduce suicide attempts.[75] Follow-up interventions are defined as services that improve access to and engagement in care as well as to prevent suicide and related behaviors.[76] This approach consists of the practice of contacting people, connecting them to care, and providing social support after discharge using phone calls, tele-assistance, or in-person visits, sending letters, emails, postcards, or caring contacts text messages.[77] In contrast to other resource intensive suicide-specific interventions that require a mental health specialist, follow-up interventions are typically brief (6–12 sessions), low cost, nondemand interventions that can be conducted by anyone and occur according to a structured schedule over a designated period (eg, 1 year).[77,78]

Although there is a paucity of randomized clinical trials on follow-up interventions for suicidal patients, existing research generally suggests that follow-up contacts may reduce repeat suicide attempts and prevent death by suicide for patients discharged from inpatient or emergency departments.[76,79,80] Specific follow-up strategies that have been shown to be effective in reducing repeat suicide attempts and/or suicide include the sending of caring letters,[81] or postcards,[82] crisis cards,[83] or short- or long-term phone or in-person contacts after hospital discharge.[84,85] Based on this evidence, the National Action Alliance for Suicide Prevention's Clinical Care and Intervention Task Force has recommended the inclusion of follow-up care for those patients at risk for suicide leaving care or transitioning from one health setting to another as one of the 4 components of evidenced based suicide prevention care.[86]

Within primary care settings, follow-up care is necessary to monitor suicide risk, connect patients to outpatient mental health specialty treatment, and promote engagement in care. Simple methods such as caring contacts and phone call contacts can easily be implemented in primary care settings by a case manager (eg, social workers nurses, psychologists) or health care assistants.[76] Another promising innovative strategy that has potential to improve access to and engagement in mental health care is the integration of care navigators into primary care settings. Care navigators, who may be clinicians, peers, or paraprofessionals, aim to support families by ensuring ongoing access to care, promoting engagement with care, facilitating shared decision making with providers, and increasing awareness of community resources.[87] Major functions and services that care navigators provide include education and coaching, advocacy, linkages to health systems and community services, and assessment and triage. While research on care navigation for pediatric populations, especially those with mental health issues or at risk for suicide, is limited, studies on adult populations with conditions like cancer or severe mental illness have shown that care navigation leads to increased health services utilization, including improved linkages to care, adherence to treatment recommendations, and timeliness in accessing health services.[88] In addition, evidence points to high patient satisfaction, enhanced understanding of diagnoses and treatments, and greater patient empowerment through navigation.[88]

Innovative Practices in Suicide Prevention in Pediatric Primary Care

The clinical pathway

Clinical pathways are tools used by health professionals to guide evidence-based practice and improve the interaction between health care professionals by adapting guidelines to a local context and detailing essential steps in assessment and treatment.[89] Clinical pathways can have positive impact on the quality of care delivered to individual patients, on the health of populations of patients with particular diseases or conditions, on the workflow of frontline providers, and on processes within the health care organization.[90,91] Suicide prevention and management strategies have been implemented by some organizations but have not been widely applied and there is a high degree of variability in care delivery across providers and settings.[92] Current estimates suggest that 30%–40% of patients do not receive treatments with proven effectiveness.[93] Within primary care, 20%–40% of adolescents have high levels of distress or suicidal ideation, yet PCPs identify less than half.[94–96] Failure to identify and intervene with youth at risk for suicide likely confers a high potential for morbidity and mortality.[97]

The clinical pathway: risk screening, assessment, and management

The clinical pathway for screening in outpatient primary care setting is depicted in **Fig. 3**. The outpatient clinical pathway was developed by the PaCC workgroup from within the Physically Ill Child committee of the AACAP to assist hospitals and emergency departments, and inpatient medical/surgical units implementing suicide risk screening to pediatric patients,[50] with subsequent versions developed for outpatient

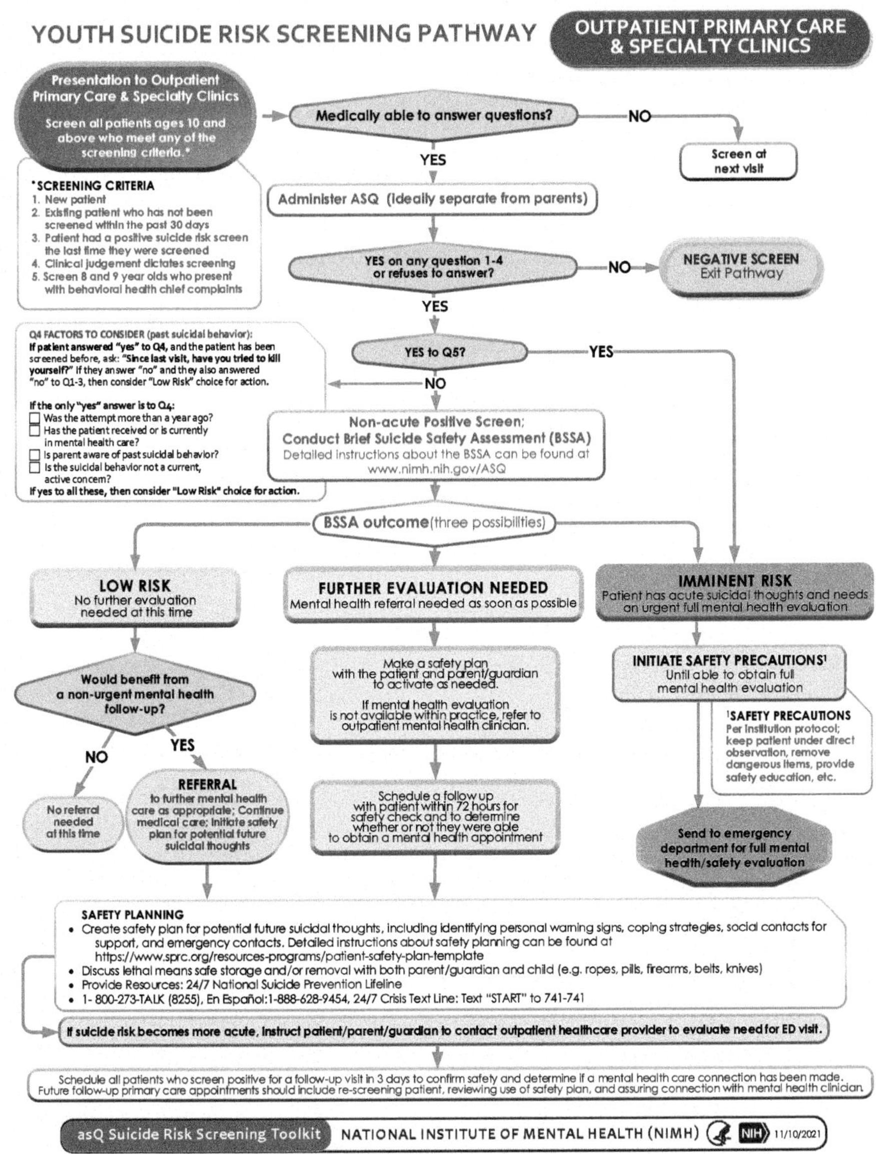

Fig. 3. Suicide risk screening pathway. Horowitz LM, Bridge JA, Tipton MV, Abernathy T, Mournet AM, Snyder DJ, Lanzillo EC, Powell D, Schoenbaum M, Brahmbhatt K, Pao M. Implementing Suicide Risk Screening in a Pediatric Primary Care Setting: From Research to Practice. Acad Pediatr. 2022 Mar;22(2):217-226. doi: 10.1016/j.acap.2021.10.012. PMID: 35248306; PMCID: PMC8908796. And can also be found at Ask Suicide-Screening Questions (ASQ) Toolkit - National Institute of Mental Health (NIMH) (nih.gov): www.nimh.nih.gov/ASQ.

primary and specialty care modified by NIMH.[98] Similar pathways have been developed for adult populations.[99] The NIMH pathway generally uses a 3-step approach to suicide risk screening (see **Fig. 2**).: (1) step 1 Brief screening for suicide risk; (2) step 2: BSSA; and step 3: determining disposition and course of action for patients deemed to be at imminent risk, in need of further evaluation or low risk for suicide.[98] The pathway was created as an evidence-informed guide to improve risk screening and effectively manage screen positive patients using the ASQ and the BSSA for screening and risk stratification (ASQ toolkit). The specific components of the clinical pathway are described later.

Step 1: Universal Screening for Suicide Risk. Universal screening for suicide risk in primary care involves screening every patient who has a primary care visit regardless of presenting complaint. The pathway is initiated by asking the child the questions on the ASQ verbatim, which takes about 20 seconds on average to complete. The initial ASQ screening should be conducted early during the primary care visit, typically at the initial nursing assessment without the parent present in the room to ensure privacy. If the child answers "no" to all ASQ questions, the screening is complete, and no further intervention is needed. If the child answers "yes" to any of questions 1 to 4, this is considered a positive screen and prompts administration of the 5th question, which captures acuity of suicide risk. If the child answers "no" to question 5, this is considered a non-acute positive screen. These patients will require further assessment using the BSSA. Answering "yes" to question 5 indicates an acute positive screen. In such instances, immediate arrangements should be made for a full mental health evaluation and safety precautions initiated.

Step 2: BSSA. The BSSA is designed to allow clinicians/providers to quickly (10–15 minutes) assess the level of suicide risk based on clinical judgment and determine if a more comprehensive mental health evaluation is needed. The BSSA should be conducted by a clinician/providers with appropriate training in suicide risk assessment.

Step 3: Developing a Disposition Plan. After completing the BSSA, the clinician determines the next action steps which are categorized into one of 3 levels of risk and discusses these recommendations with the patients and parents or guardian.

1. *Low Risk*: A low risk BSSA outcome indicates that no further evaluation is needed at this time. Depending upon the circumstances, some patients may benefit from a non-urgent mental health follow-up referral. For patients referred for mental health care, a safety plan should be created with the child and/or parent/guardian for potential future suicidal thoughts. The recommended standard of care would be to provide the patient and parent or guardian basic safety education (eg, lethal means safe storage and removal), education about warning signs for suicide, and crisis resources.
2. *Moderate Risk: Further evaluation is Needed.* A moderate risk BSSA result indicates that further mental health evaluation is needed as soon as possible. If a mental health evaluation is not available within the primary care practice, the patient should be referred to an outpatient mental health specialty clinic or crisis intervention service. As part of the mental health evaluation, a safety plan should be developed with the patient and family and lethal means safe storage and removal should be discussed. Patients should also receive follow-up care within 72 hours of the initial visit for a safety check and to determine whether or not they were able to obtain a mental health appointment. Patients should also be given crisis resources such as the National Suicide Lifeline and the crisis text line upon discharge home.
3. *Imminent Risk:* Patients at imminent risk have acute suicidal thoughts and need an urgent full mental health evaluation. Safety precautions (eg, keeping the patient under direct observation removing dangerous items) should be initiated within the primary care practice and the patient should be sent to the emergency department for a full mental health/safety evaluation. It should be noted that less than 1% of youth who present to primary care settings are at imminent risk for suicide.[98]

The clinical pathway: follow-up and continuity of care

Follow-up care both within and outside the primary care clinic is essential for patients who screen positive for suicide risk to ensure continuity of care and prevent future suicide behavior and suicide. As previously discussed (see section on follow-up and monitoring), caring contacts (including following up phone calls or texts within 72 hours of the initial visit) can be an effective strategy for reducing suicidal behavior. Other linkage/bridging strategies such as contacting the outpatient mental health provider to provide a warm handoff can also help to ensure continuity of care.

Educating pediatric primary care providers in suicide prevention

Despite being at the forefront of suicide prevention, recent surveys suggest that PCPs often lack adequate training in suicide prevention and intervention strategies.[100–102] Research highlights that properly training primary care doctors and nurses can significantly lower rates of suicide, non-fatal suicide attempts, and suicidal thoughts.[70] This underscores the importance of expanding training opportunities for PCPs. It is essential that pediatric residency programs and continuing medical education events integrate curricula focused on assessing and managing youth suicide risk. These training opportunities should teach PCPs how to engage in validating, effective, and non-stigmatizing conversations with at-risk patients, utilize validated and evidence-based screening tools, and apply best practices such as safety planning and lethal means counseling.[100] Additionally, training should cover how to connect patients with community resources to ensure continuous support.

Collaborative care models

Collaborative care models (CCMs) in primary care are increasingly recognized as effective approaches for addressing suicide risk, particularly due to their integrated, team-based nature that enhances the delivery of mental health care. CCMs are comprehensive, system level interventions that restructure care delivery. These models optimize efficiency by connecting PCPs and patients with mental health specialists to enhance evidence-based treatment for mental health disorders.[103] Care managers play a vital role in coordinating interventions, supporting decision-making and communication between the patient and the PCP, monitoring mental health symptoms and medication use, and ensuring treatment adherence.[103]

Although no studies have evaluated the effectiveness of CCM on suicidal behaviors in pediatric populations, research on older adults has shown that CCMs can significantly reduce suicidal ideation and symptoms of depression.[104,105] Additionally, several randomized controlled trials focusing on adolescents with depression in primary care settings have demonstrated the effectiveness of CCMs in decreasing depression and improving adherence to evidenced-base treatments.[106–109]

SUMMARY

Suicide among youth represents a significant public health challenge, and primary care providers are crucial in addressing this issue. Key strategies for prevention in primary care include using validated tools for suicide risk screening, conducting comprehensive assessments, and implementing brief interventions like safety planning. Continuous follow-up and monitoring are also essential. Additionally, CCMs have been shown to be effective in reducing suicidal ideation and attempts by integrating behavioral health services with primary care. The NIMH Clinical Pathway offers an innovative framework for incorporating these interventions, but the effectiveness of such strategies depends heavily on the training and preparedness of clinicians. By investing in comprehensive and ongoing training, the health care system can better equip primary care providers to manage this critical aspect of youth health effectively. Future studies are also needed to test the effectiveness of the clinical pathway within primary care settings.

CLINICS CARE POINTS

- Suicide Prevention Resource Center https://sprc.org/settings/.
- Zero Suicide https://zerosuicide.edc.org.
- Ask Suicide Screening Questions (ASQ) https://www.nimh.nih.gov/research/research-conducted-at-nimh/asq-toolkit-materials.

ACKNOWLEDGMENTS

This work was supported by grant 5P50MH127476 from the National Institute of Mental Health, United States (Drs J.A. Bridge and C.A. Fontanella, Co-PIs).

DISCLOSURE

The authors have nothing to disclose.

REFERENCES

1. Centers for Disease Control and Prevention, Web-based Injury Statistics Query and Reporting System (WISQARS) Leading Cause of Death [online]. National Center for Injury Prevention and Control. Available at: https://wisqars.cdc.gov/lcd/?o=LCD&y1=2021&y2=2021&ct=10&cc=. (Accessed April 7 2024).
2. Centers for Disease Control and Prevention. Web-based Injury Statistics Query and Reporting System (WISQARS) Fatal Death Reports [online]. National Center for Injury Prevention and Control. Available at: https://webappa.cdc.gov/sasweb/ncipc/mortrate.html. (Accessed April 12 2024).
3. O'Carroll PW, Berman AL, Maris RW, et al. Beyond the tower of Babel: A nomenclature for suicidology. Suicide Life-Threatening Behav 1996;26(3):237–52.
4. Centers for Disease Control and Prevention. Youth risk behavior survey data summary & trends report: 2011 - 2021 2023. Available at: https://www.cdc.gov/healthyyouth/data/yrbs/pdf/YRBS_Data-Summary-Trends_Report2023_508.pdf. (Accessed April 13 2024).
5. Campo JV. Youth suicide prevention: Does access to care matter? Curr Opin Pediatr 2009;21(5):628–34.
6. Green C, Gottschlich EA, Burr WH. A national survey of pediatricians' experiences and practices with suicide prevention. Acad Pediatr 2023;23(7):1403–10.
7. Ahmedani BK, Simon GE, Stewart C, et al. Health care contacts in the year before suicide death. J Gen Intern Med 2014;29(6):870–7.
8. Luoma JB, Martin CE, Pearson JL. Contact with mental health and primary care providers before suicide: A review of the evidence. Am J Psychiatr 2002;159(6):909–16.
9. Andrilla CHA, Patterson DG, Garberson LA, et al. Geographic variation in the supply of selected behavioral health providers. Am J Prev Med 2018;54(6):S199–207.

10. Cummings JR, Allen L, Clennon J, et al. Geographic access to specialty mental health care across high- and low-income US communities. JAMA Psychiatr 2017;74(5):476.
11. Shain B, Braverman PK, Adelman WP, et al. Suicide and Suicide Attempts in Adolescents. Pediatrics 2016;138(1):e20161420–2016.
12. Cha CB, Franz PJ, E MG, et al. Annual research review: Suicide among youth - epidemiology, (potential) etiology, and treatment. J Child Psychol Psychiatry 2018;59(4):460–82.
13. Ruch DA, Sheftall AH, Schlagbaum P, et al. Trends in Suicide Among Youth Aged 10 to 19 Years in the United States, 1975 to 2016. JAMA Netw Open 2019;2(5):e193886.
14. Bridge JA, Horowitz LM, Fontanella CA, et al. Age-related racial disparity in suicide rates among US youths from 2001 through 2015. JAMA Pediatr 2018; 172(7):697–9.
15. Raifman J, Charlton BM, Arrington-Sanders R, et al. Sexual orientation and suicide attempt disparities among US Adolescents: 2009–2017. Pediatrics 2020; 145(3):e20191658.
16. Horowitz LM, Mournet AM, Lanzillo E, et al. Screening pediatric medical patients for suicide risk: Is depression screening enough? J Adolesc Health 2021;68(6): 1183–8.
17. Perou R, Bitsko RH, Blumberg SJ, et al. Mental health surveillance among children–United States, 2005-2011. MMWR Suppl 2013;62(2):1–35.
18. Ghandour RM, Sherman LJ, Vladutiu CJ, et al. Prevalence and treatment of depression, anxiety, and conduct problems in US children. J Pediatr 2019; 206:256–67.e3.
19. Czyz EK, King CA. Longitudinal trajectories of suicidal ideation and subsequent suicide attempts among adolescent inpatients. J Clin Child Adolesc Psychol 2015;44(1):181–93.
20. SAMHSA, National survey on drug use and health (NSDUH) 2023. Available at: https://www.samhsa.gov/data/release/2022-national-survey-drug-use-and-health-nsduh-releases, (Accessed May 3 2024). 2022.
21. Goldston DB, Daniel SS, Erkanli A, et al. Psychiatric diagnoses as contemporaneous risk factors for suicide attempts among adolescents and young adults: Developmental changes. J Consult Clin Psychol 2009;77(2):281–90.
22. Brent DA, Melhem NM, Oquendo M, et al. Familial pathways to early-onset suicide attempt: A 5.6-year prospective study. JAMA Psychiatr 2015;72(2):160–8.
23. DeVille DC, Whalen D, Breslin FJ, et al. Prevalence and family-related factors associated with suicidal ideation, suicide attempts, and self-injury in children aged 9 to 10 years. JAMA Netw Open 2020;3(2):e1920956.
24. Timmons KA, Selby EA, Lewinsohn PM, et al. Parental displacement and adolescent suicidality: Exploring the role of failed belonging. J Clin Child Adolesc Psychol 2011;40(6):807–17.
25. Angelakis I, Austin JL, Gooding P. Association of childhood maltreatment with suicide behaviors among young people: A systematic review and meta-analysis. JAMA Netw Open 2020;3(8):e2012563.
26. Gomez SH, Tse J, Wang Y, et al. Are there sensitive periods when child maltreatment substantially elevates suicide risk? Results from a nationally representative sample of adolescents. Depress Anxiety 2017;34(8):734–41.
27. Koyanagi A, Oh H, Carvalho AF, et al. Bullying victimization and suicide attempt among adolescents aged 12-15 years From 48 countries. J Am Acad Child Adolesc Psychiatry 2019;58(9):907–18.e4.

28. Alavi N, Reshetukha T, Prost E, et al. Relationship between bullying and suicidal behaviour in youth presenting to the emergency department. J Can Acad Child Adolesc Psychiatry 2017;26(2):70–7.
29. Mueller AS, Abrutyn S. Suicidal disclosures among friends: Using social network data to understand suicide contagion. J Health Soc Behav 2015;56(1):131–48.
30. Katz C, Bolton SL, Katz LY, et al, Swampy Cree Suicide Prevention Team. A systematic review of school-based suicide prevention programs. Research Support, Non-U.S. Gov't Review. Depress Anxiety 2013;30(10):1030–45.
31. Singer J, Erbacher T, Rosen P. School-based suicide prevention: A framework for evidence-based practice. School Mental Health 2019;11. https://doi.org/10.1007/s12310-018-9245-8.
32. Sedgwick R, Epstein S, Dutta R, et al. Social media, internet use and suicide attempts in adolescents. Curr Opin Psychiatry 2019;32(6):534–41.
33. Marchant A, Hawton K, Stewart A, et al. A systematic review of the relationship between internet use, self-harm and suicidal behaviour in young people: The good, the bad and the unknown. PLoS One 2017;12(8):e0181722.
34. Niederkrotenthaler T, Braun M, Pirkis J, et al. Association between suicide reporting in the media and suicide: Systematic review and meta-analysis. BMJ 2020;m575. https://doi.org/10.1136/bmj.m575.
35. Bridge JA, Greenhouse JB, Ruch D, et al. Association between the release of Netflix's 13 Reasons Why and suicide rates in the United States: An interrupted time series analysis. J Am Acad Child Adolesc Psychiatry 2020;59(2):236–43.
36. Allgaier A-K, Pietsch K, Frühe B, et al. Screening for depression in adolescents: Validity of the patient health questionnaire in pediatriv care. Depress Anxiety 2012;29(10):906–13.
37. Richardson LP, McCauley E, Grossman DC, et al. Evaluation of the Patient Health Questionnaire-9 Item for detecting major depression among adolescents. Pediatrics 2010;126(6):1117–23.
38. Kemper AR, Hostutler CA, Beck K, et al. Depression and suicide-risk screening results in pediatric primary care. Pediatrics 2021. https://doi.org/10.1542/peds.2021-049999.
39. Aguinaldo LD, Sullivant S, Lanzillo EC, et al. Validation of the ask suicide-screening questions (ASQ) with youth in outpatient specialty and primary care clinics. Gen Hosp Psychiatry 2021;68:52–8.
40. Horowitz LM, Bridge JA, Teach SJ, et al. Ask Suicide-Screening Questions (ASQ): A brief instrument for the pediatric emergency department. Arch Pediatr Adolesc Med 2012;166(12):1170–6.
41. Ballard ED, Cwik M, Van Eck K, et al. Identification of at-risk youth by suicide screening in a pediatric emergency department. Prev Sci 2017;18(2):174–82.
42. DeVylder JE, Ryan TC, Cwik M, et al. Assessment of selective and universal screening for suicide risk in a pediatric emergency department. JAMA Netw Open 2019;2(10):e1914070.
43. Reynolds W, Mazza J. Assessment of suicidal ideation in inner-city children and young adolescents: Reliability and validity of the Suicidal Ideation Questionnaire-JR. Sch Psychol Rev 1999;28. https://doi.org/10.1080/02796015.1999.12085945.
44. Hetrick SE, Gao CX, Filia KM, et al. Validation of a brief tool to assess and monitor suicidal ideation: The Youth Suicide Ideation Screen (YSIS-3). J Affect Disord 2021;295:235–42.

45. Mayes TL, Kennard BD, Killian M, et al. Psychometric properties of the concise health risk tracking (CHRT) in adolescents with suicidality. J Affect Disord 2018; 235:45–51.
46. Hughes JL, Horowitz LM, Ackerman JP, et al. Suicide in young people: Screening, risk assessment, and intervention. BMJ 2023;381:e070630.
47. Busby DR, Hughes JL, Walters M, et al. Measurement choices for youth suicidality. Child Psychiatry Hum Dev 2023. https://doi.org/10.1007/s10578-023-01627-5.
48. Christensen LeCloux M, Aguinaldo LD, Lanzillo EC, et al. Provider opinions of the acceptability of Ask Suicide-Screening Questions (ASQ) Tool and the ASQ Brief Suicide Safety Assessment (BSSA) for universal suicide risk screening in community healthcare: Potential barriers and necessary elements for future implementation. J Behav Health Serv Res 2022;49(3):346–63.
49. Snyder DJ, Jordan BA, Aizvera J, et al. From pilot to practice: Implementation of a suicide risk screening program in hospitalized medical patients. Jt Comm J Qual Patient Saf 2020;46(7):417–26.
50. Brahmbhatt K, Kurtz BP, Afzal KI, et al. Suicide risk screening in pediatric hospitals: clinical pathways to address a global health crisis. Psychosomatics 2019; 60(1):1–9.
51. Molock SD, Boyd RC, Alvarez K, et al. Culturally responsive assessment of suicidal thoughts and behaviors in youth of color. Am Psychol 2023;78(7):842–55.
52. DeCrane O, Zhang J, Parrott B, et al. "Where are the pediatricians in all this?": Family perspectives on the role of pediatricians in mental healthcare and suicide prevention. SSM Ment Health 2024;5. https://doi.org/10.1016/j.ssmmh.2024.100307.
53. Asarnow JR, Baraff LJ, Berk M, et al. An emergency department intervention for linking pediatric suicidal patients to follow-up mental health treatment. Psychiatr Serv 2011;62(11):1303–9.
54. Hughes JL, Asarnow JR. Enhanced mental health interventions in the emergency department: Suicide and suicide attempt prevention in the ED. Clin Pediatr Emerg Med 2013;14(1):28–34.
55. Nuij C, van Ballegooijen W, de Beurs D, et al. Safety planning-type interventions for suicide prevention: Meta-analysis. Br J Psychiatry 2021;219(2):419–26.
56. McCabe R, Garside R, Backhouse A, et al. Effectiveness of brief psychological interventions for suicidal presentations: a systematic review. BMC Psychiatr 2018; 18(1):120.
57. Czyz EK, King CA, Biermann BJ. Motivational interviewing-enhanced safety planning for adolescents at high suicide risk: A pilot randomized controlled trial. J Clin Child Adolesc Psychol 2019;48(2):250–62.
58. Micol VJ, Prouty D, Czyz EK. Enhancing motivation and self-efficacy for safety plan use: Incorporating motivational interviewing strategies in a brief safety planning intervention for adolescents at risk for suicide. Psychotherapy 2022; 59(2):174–80.
59. Chesin MS, Stanley B, Haigh EA, et al. Staff views of an emergency department intervention using safety planning and structured follow-up with suicidal veterans. Arch Suicide Res 2017;21(1):127–37.
60. Stanley B, Brown G, Brent DA, et al. Cognitive-behavioral therapy for suicide prevention (CBT-SP): Treatment model, feasibility, and acceptability. J Am Acad Child Adolesc Psychiatry 2009;48(10):1005–13.
61. Stanley B, Brown GK. Safety planning intervention: A brief intervention to mitigate suicide risk. Cognit Behav Pract 2012;19(2):256–64.

62. Brent DA, Greenhill LL, Compton S, et al. The treatment of adolescent suicide attempters study (TASA): Predictors of suicidal events in an open treatment trial. J Am Acad Child Adolesc Psychiatry 2009;48(10):987–96.
63. Stanley B, Brown GK, Brenner LA, et al. Comparison of the safety planning intervention with follow-up vs usual care of suicidal patients treated in the emergency department. JAMA Psychiatr 2018;75(9):894–900.
64. Adrian M, McCauley E, Gallop R, et al. Advancing suicide intervention strategies for teens (ASSIST): Study protocol for a multisite randomised controlled trial. BMJ Open 2023;13(12):e074116.
65. Asarnow JR, Berk M, Hughes JL, et al. The SAFETY program: A treatment-development trial of a cognitive-behavioral family treatment for adolescent suicide attempters. J Clin Child Adolesc Psychol 2015;44(1):194–203.
66. Asarnow JR, Hughes J, Cohen D, et al. The incubator treatment development model: The SAFETY treatment for suicidal/self-harming youth. Cognit Behav Pract 2022;29(1):185–97.
67. Asarnow JR, Hughes JL, Babeva KN, et al. Cognitive-behavioral family treatment for suicide attempt prevention: A randomized controlled trial. J Am Acad Child Adolesc Psychiatry 2017;56(6):506–14.
68. Hughes JL, Asarnow JR. Implementing and adapting the SAFETY treatment for suicidal youth: The incubator model, telehealth, and the Covid-19 pandemic. Cognit Behav Pract 2022;29(1):198–213.
69. Rotheram-Borus MJ, Piacentini J, Van Rossem R, et al. Enhancing treatment adherence with a specialized emergency room program for adolescent suicide attempters. J Am Acad Child Adolesc Psychiatry 1996;35(5):654–63.
70. Mann JJ, Michel CA, Auerbach RP. Improving Suicide Prevention Through Evidence-Based Strategies: A Systematic Review. Am J Psychiatry 2021;178(7): 611–24.
71. Kruesi MJ, Grossman J, Pennington JM, et al. Suicide and violence prevention: Parent education in the emergency department. J Am Acad Child Adolesc Psychiatry 1999;38(3):250–5.
72. Bandealy A, Herrera N, Weissman M, et al. Use of lethal means restriction counseling for suicide prevention in pediatric primary care. Prev Med 2020;130: 105855.
73. American Academy of Pediatrics. American Foundation for Suicide Prevention. National Institute of Mental Health. Suicide: Blueprint for Youth Suicide Prevention. Available at: https://www.aap.org/en/patient-care/blueprint-for-youth-suicide-prevention/. (Accessed April 4 2024).
74. Asarnow JR, Zullo L, Ernestus SM, et al. "Lock and Protect": Development of a Digital Decision Aid to Support Lethal Means Counseling in Parents of Suicidal Youth. Front Psychiatry 2021;12:736236.
75. Zalsman G, Hawton K, Wasserman D, et al. Suicide prevention strategies revisited: 10-year systematic review. Lancet Psychiatr 2016;3(7):646–59.
76. Brown GK, Green KL. A review of evidence-based follow-up care for suicide prevention: Where do we go from here? Am J Prev Med 2014;47(3 Suppl 2):S209–15.
77. Milner AJ, Carter G, Pirkis J, et al. Letters, green cards, telephone calls and postcards: Systematic and meta-analytic review of brief contact interventions for reducing self-harm, suicide attempts and suicide. Br J Psychiatry 2015; 206(3):184–90.
78. Stanley B, Brodsky B, Monahan M. Brief and ultra-brief suicide-specific interventions. FOCUS 2023;21(2):129–36.

79. Luxton DD, June JD, Comtois KA. Can postdischarge follow-up contacts prevent suicide and suicidal behavior? Crisis 2013;34(1):32–41.
80. Ghanbari B, Malakouti SK, Nojomi M, et al. Suicide prevention and follow-up services: A narrative review. Global J Health Sci 2015;8(5):145.
81. Motto JA, Bostrom AG. A randomized controlled trial of postcrisis suicide prevention. Psychiatr Serv 2001;52(6):828–33.
82. Carter GL, Clover K, Whyte IM, et al. Postcards from the EDge: 5-year outcomes of a randomised controlled trial for hospital-treated self-poisoning. Br J Psychiatry 2013;202(5):372–80.
83. Kapur N, Cooper J, Bennewith O, et al. Postcards, green cards and telephone calls: Therapeutic contact with individuals following self-harm. Br J Psychiatry 2010;197(1):5–7.
84. Fleischmann A, Bertolote JM, Wasserman D, et al. Effectiveness of brief intervention and contact for suicide attempters: a randomized controlled trial in five countries. Bull World Health Organ 2008;86(9):703–9.
85. Vaiva G, Vaiva G, Ducrocq F, et al. Effect of telephone contact on further suicide attempts in patients discharged from an emergency department: Randomised controlled study. Bmj 2006;332(7552):1241–5.
86. Covington D, Hogan M, Abreu J, et al. Suicide care in systems framework. National Action Alliance. Clinical Care & Intervention Task Force 2011.
87. McDonald KM, Sundaram V, Bravata DM, et al. Closing the quality gap: a critical analysis of quality improvement strategies (vol. 7: care Coordination). Rockville, MD: Agency for Healthcare Research and Quality (US); 2007.
88. Godoy L, Hodgkinson S, Robertson HA, et al. Increasing mental health engagement from primary care: The potential role of family navigation. Pediatrics 2019; 143(4):e20182418.
89. Kinsman L, Rotter T, James E, et al. What is a clinical pathway? Development of a definition to inform the debate. BMC Med 2010;8:31.
90. Rotter T, Kinsman L, Machotta A, et al. Clinical pathways for primary care: effects on professional practice, patient outcomes, and costs. Cochrane Database Syst Rev 2013;(8). https://doi.org/10.1002/14651858.CD010706.
91. Rotter T, Kinsman L, James E, et al. Clinical pathways: Effects on professional practice, patient outcomes, length of stay and hospital costs. Cochrane Database Syst Rev 2010;(3):Cd006632.
92. Hogan MF, Grumet JG. Suicide prevention: An emerging priority for health care. Health Aff 2016;35(6):1084–90.
93. Agency for Healthcare Research and Quality. 2019 National Healthcare Quality and Disparities Report. Available at: https://www.ahrq.gov/research/findings/nhqrdr/nhqdr19/index.html/. (Accessed April 13 2024).
94. Ozer EM, Zahnd EG, Adams SH, et al. Are adolescents being screened for emotional distress in primary care? J Adolesc Health 2009;44(6):520–7.
95. McKelvey RS, Davies LC, Pfaff JJ, et al. Psychological distress and suicidal ideation among 15-24-year-olds presenting to general practice: A pilot study. Aust N Z J Psychiatry 1998;32(3):344–8.
96. Pfaff JJ, Acres JG, McKelvey RS. Training general practitioners to recognise and respond to psychological distress and suicidal ideation in young people. Med J Aust 2001;174(5):222–6.
97. Bridge JA, Goldstein TR, Brent DA. Adolescent suicide and suicidal behavior. JCPP (J Child Psychol Psychiatry) 2006;47(3–4):372–94.

98. Horowitz LM, Bridge JA, Tipton MV, et al. Implementing suicide risk screening in a pediatric primary care setting: From research to practice. Acad Pediatr 2022; 22(2):217–26.
99. Ayer L, Horowitz LM, Colpe L, et al. Clinical pathway for suicide risk screening in adult primary care settings: Special recommendations. J Acad Consult Liaison Psychiatry 2022;63(5):497–510.
100. Schoen LE, Bogetz AL, Hom MA, et al. Suicide risk assessment and management training practices in pediatric residency programs: A nationwide needs assessment survey. J Adolesc Health 2019;65(2):280–8.
101. Sudak D, Roy A, Sudak H, et al. Deficiencies in suicide training in primary care specialties: A survey of training directors. Acad Psychiatry 2007;31(5):345–9.
102. Hawgood JL, Krysinska KE, Ide N, et al. Is suicide prevention properly taught in medical schools? Med Teach 2008;30(3):287–95.
103. Goodrich DE, Kilbourne AM, Nord KM, et al. Mental health collaborative care and its role in primary care settings. Curr Psychiatr Rep 2013;15(8).
104. Bruce ML, Ten Have TR, Reynolds CF 3rd, et al. Reducing suicidal ideation and depressive symptoms in depressed older primary care patients: A randomized controlled trial. JAMA 2004;291(9):1081–91.
105. Unützer J, Tang L, Oishi S, et al. Reducing suicidal ideation in depressed older primary care patients. J Am Geriatr Soc 2006;54(10):1550–6.
106. Richardson LP, Ludman E, McCauley E, et al. Collaborative care for adolescents with depression in primary care. JAMA 2014;312(8):809.
107. Asarnow JR, Jaycox LH, Duan N, et al. Effectiveness of a quality improvement intervention for adolescent dpression in primary care clinics. JAMA 2005;293(3):311.
108. Wells KB, Tang L, Carlson GA, et al. Treatment of youth depression in primary care under usual practice conditions: Observational findings from youth partners in care. J Child Adolesc Psychopharmacol 2012;22(1):80–90.
109. Asarnow JR, Jaycox LH, Tang L, et al. Long-term benefits of short-term quality improvement interventions for depressed youths in primary care. Am J Psychiatr 2009;166(9):1002–10.

Addressing Mental Health and Social Needs in Tandem to Promote Health Equity

Chidiogo Anyigbo, MD, MPH[a,b,*], Sarah J. Beal, PhD[a,b,c], Joyce Y. Lee, PhD[d], Laura M. Gottlieb, MD, MPH[e,f]

KEYWORDS

• Social determinants of health • Social risk • Social need • Mental health • Intersectionality • Social care delivery

KEY POINTS

- Substantial evidence supports associations between social risks and mental health outcomes.
- To maximize the effectiveness of interventions that prevent or treat mental health concerns, screening for social risks and social needs should be administered in tandem with screening for mental health concerns.
- Family functioning plays a key role in addressing both children's mental health and their families' and caregivers' social needs.
- Equipping families to address both social and mental health needs should involve coordinated, multi-sectoral partnerships and interventions.

CHILD AND YOUTH MENTAL HEALTH IS IN CRISIS

Both the Surgeon General and the American Academy of Pediatrics have called attention to the national mental health crisis, which impacts young people and their caregivers, acknowledging that child and youth mental health and parental mental

[a] Division of General and Community Pediatrics, Cincinnati Children's Hospital Medical Center, 3333 Burnet Avenue, MLC 7035, Cincinnati, OH 45229, USA; [b] Department of Pediatrics, College of Medicine, University of Cincinnati, Cincinnati, OH, USA; [c] Behavioral Medicine and Clinical Psychology, Division of General and Community Pediatrics, Cincinnati Children's Hospital Medical Center, 3333 Burnet Avenue, MLC 7039, Cincinnati, OH 45229, USA; [d] College of Social Work, The Ohio State University, Stillman Hall 225C, 1947 North College Road, Columbus, OH 43210, USA; [e] Department of Family and Community Medicine, University of California, San Francisco, CA, USA; [f] Social Interventions Research and Evaluation Network, University of California, 5th Floor, 675 18th Street, San Francisco, CA 94107, USA
* Corresponding author.
E-mail address: chidiogo.anyigbo@cchmc.org
Twitter: @CincyChildrens (C.A.); @CFWlaboratory (S.J.B.); @joyceyeaeunlee (J.Y.L.); @SIREN_UCSF (L.M.G.)

Pediatr Clin N Am 71 (2024) 1141–1149
https://doi.org/10.1016/j.pcl.2024.07.018 pediatric.theclinics.com

health impact well-being across the lifespan.[1,2] 20% of youth ages 3 to 17 years have some type of mental health problem. This includes a recent rise in major depressive episodes in youth and increased pediatric suicidal thoughts, attempts, and completions. Suicide is now the third most common cause of death in young people aged 15 to 24 years and second most common cause for youth aged 10 to 14 years.[3]

Mental health challenges in childhood and adolescence can have lifelong effects. Approximately 50% of adults with mental health challenges experienced onset in childhood or adolescence.[4,5] Mental health affects how young people view themselves, their relationships, and their academic and professional trajectories. Experiences with mental health challenges in childhood can pose lifelong barriers to health.[6,7] This makes early intervention critical to long-term health optimization.

Improving child and adolescent mental health requires multi-sectoral solutions. The US Surgeon General's Advisory on the youth mental health crisis outlines the many efforts various sectors of society can undertake in addressing youth mental health.[8] This includes roles for health care teams that serve this population, such as in screening children and youth for mental health risk factors and challenges. The Surgeon General also explicitly calls for assessing and addressing not only mental health needs but also the other needs of caregivers and family members.[8]

This paper calls attention to and broadens the scope of the Surgeon General's instruction to assess and address youth mental health alongside the other needs of caregivers and families as a strategy for improving child and adolescent mental health.

UNADDRESSED SOCIAL RISK FACTORS EXACERBATE THE PEDIATRIC MENTAL HEALTH CRISIS

The US child and adolescent mental health crisis is exacerbated by the inequitable societal distribution of power and resources and the social conditions that stem from that distribution, conditions such as the availability of healthy food, safe housing, steady employment, and reliable transportation. Access to these types of material resources can affect family and patient functioning and has been consistently associated with mental health outcomes.[9,10] In pediatrics, social risk factors must be viewed in the context of familial and household relationships because children rely on adult caregivers who are also experiencing the direct effects of social risk factors. For example, food insecurity can affect emotional regulation. Additionally, the stress adult caregivers experience due to food insecurity may deplete caregivers' emotional resources to provide effective emotional co-regulation support to their children, worsening emotional dysregulation.[11,12] This compounding effect means that pediatric clinicians must consider the social needs of all family members when addressing the specific mental health needs of a single pediatric patient.

The impact of social risk factors on mental health symptoms manifests in different ways across child development. For example, household social risk factors (eg, poverty, food insecurity) are associated with emotional dysregulation in early childhood,[13] with health risk behaviors such as substance use in adolescence,[14] which influences outcomes such as education and employment in adulthood.[15] Succinctly, family-level social needs can contribute both to dysregulation and associated internalizing and externalizing symptoms that contribute to mental health risk across the lifespan.[16,17]

The interplay between social context and mental health in the United States also leads to profound inequities in mental health across multiple demographic groups. For instance, there are higher rates of suicide among youth of color and those with minoritized sexual orientation and gender identities.[3,18] Higher rates of mental health challenges are also associated with lower socioeconomic status, experiencing precarious employment, financial hardship, and having unmet basic needs such as food insecurity.[19,20]

IT IS CRITICAL TO ADDRESS MENTAL HEALTH AND SOCIAL NEEDS IN TANDEM

Integrating Social Care into Mental Health Care

Social needs and mental health are closely interwoven; therefore, integrating mental health screening and treatment into pediatric care delivery is necessary but insufficient to address the pediatric mental health crisis in the United States. Mental health screening must be accompanied by social risk screening and interventions.[21] Not surprisingly, the benefits of integrated care are likely to be reciprocal: improved social conditions will influence mental health and improved mental health will influence social conditions.

The Social Interventions Research and Evaluation Network Social Care Logic Model (**Fig. 1**) illustrates multiple mechanisms through which addressing families' social needs might influence health outcomes.[22] When applied to pediatric mental health, the model points to the different pathways through which screening and addressing social needs can affect children's mental health, including by increasing connections with both social and mental health services, strengthening patients' and caregivers' emotional supports, and promoting disease self-management. Supporting families in seeing ways to concurrently address social needs and their children's mental health concerns is an important step to ensure improved child health and well-being.

Since pediatric primary care settings are not uniformly resourced and the level of need will vary across settings, clinic context will affect the ways in which social and mental health can be integrated. At a minimum, settings serving children should consider adding workflows to facilitate both social and mental health screening into their clinical practices to identify unmet mental and social needs. The American Academy of Pediatrics Screening Technical Assistance and Resource Center[23] provides a screening tool finder that includes both mental health and social risk assessment tools that can support clinical teams to find the appropriate instruments.

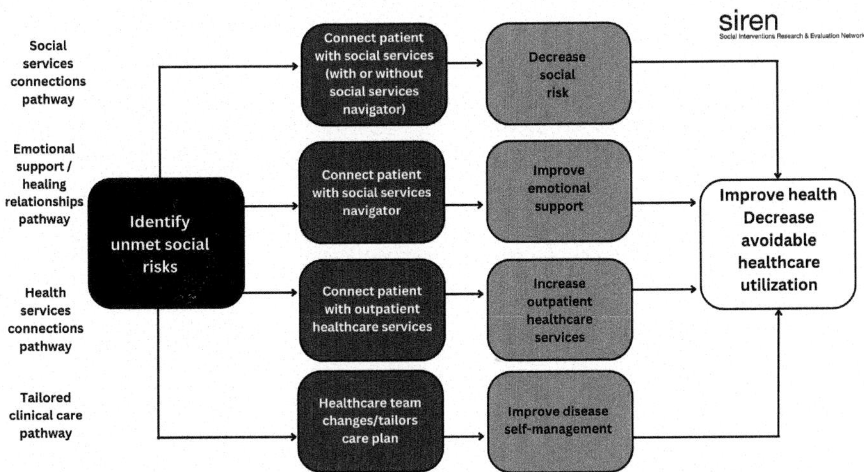

Fig. 1. Social interventions research and evaluation network social care logic model. (Gottlieb, et al., "Revising the Logic Model Behind Health Care's Social Care Investments." *Milbank Quarterly.* 2024.)

A subsequent challenge is implementing and sustaining effective interventions. Some best practice models co-locate or ideally, integrate behavioral health interventions and social service referrals and navigation supports. Integration demands intentional coordination and harmonization across these programs. We present 2 cases below that highlight possible integrated approaches to mental and social health care.

Case Examples of Integrated Mental and Social Health Care in Clinical Practice

Case 1

Scenario

A mother presents for their infant's 4-mo well-child visit with a concern of increased fussiness after missing the 2-mo well-child visit. As part of the clinical practice, a comprehensive screening includes an Edinburgh Postpartum Depression Scale (EPDS) and social risk screening. The mother reports food insecurity and transportation insecurity on the social risk screening and postpartum depression (PPD) on the EPDS.

Integrated Care Approach

- Clinician and the mother discuss interconnections between the unmet basic needs and PPD and the infant's fussiness. The clinician underscores the clinic's commitment to addressing both mental and social health needs as part of comprehensive care.
- Clinician and the mother discuss the mother's priorities around addressing identified needs.
- Parent expresses interest in support addressing food needs. She also would like to explore telehealth as an option for follow-up visits for PPD so that transportation will not pose a barrier to care.
- The clinician makes referral to a behavioral health specialist for mother's PPD. The behavioral health specialist is aware of the steps being taken to address families' social needs and understands accommodations that may be needed re: scheduling around transportation availability.

Case 2

Scenario

A father brings his 5-year-old and 7-year-old children to the clinic complaining that for the last 3 months both children have had difficulty sleeping, often have nightmares, and have been repeatedly accused of disrupting their classrooms. When asked about the household sleep routine, the father reports a 6-month history of housing insecurity that has involved sleeping on several friends' couches. He is concerned they may soon need to move into a homeless shelter.

Integrated Care Approach

- Clinician and the father discuss the connection between housing instability, sleep disturbances, and the children's behavioral challenges at school.
- The clinician recognizes the difficulty of addressing sleep challenges in the setting of precarious housing and focuses the discussion on what the father feels is realistic for improving his children's sleep schedule.
- Clinician makes a social work referral to explore options for more stable family housing.
- Clinician and the father discuss initiating a brief bedtime routine he believes would be realistic in different settings.

Key clinic implementation considerations when addressing mental health and social needs in pediatric primary care settings include.

- Elevating the intersection of social needs and mental health concerns and treatment options.
- Understanding the local setting's resources, including human capital, technology capacity, and community resource availability.
- Selecting screening tools to assess family strengths, social and mental health risks, and family priorities.

- Using trauma-informed principles to ensure care is guided by the family's priorities.
- Engaging strategies that leverage the skills and strengths of the clinicians, ancillary staff, social workers, and community health workers.

The workforce, technology, and other resources needed to meaningfully implement and sustain integrated interventions will require multi-sector partnerships. These partnerships can help health care systems access financial resources for new staff and programs, contribute to policy change, and equitably allocate critical resources.[24–29]

Potential partners might include.

- Families and caregivers with relevant lived experience to inform the development and implementation of processes to best meet family needs.
- Community organizations that provide services to address social needs and mental health needs.
- Health care payors to support the integration of social care and mental health interventions.
- Early learning centers and schools.
- Local city leaders and local government.
- Collaborations with those who can provide digital and technology resources.

THE IMPORTANCE OF WORKING WITH FAMILIES AND CREATING ANTI-RACIST CARE SYSTEMS TO ADDRESS MENTAL HEALTH AND SOCIAL NEEDS

Even with integrated care workflow and meaningful interventions to address social and mental health needs, pediatric clinics and systems will continuously face threats to equitable social and mental health care. These threats are a result of 2 systemically-created challenges.

First is the child-centric focus inherent the discipline of pediatrics that often leads to the separation of child social and mental health needs from caregivers' and families' social and mental health needs. Pediatric clinicians and practices must recognize that addressing caregivers' and families' social and mental health needs is part of treating children's mental health concerns. As previously stated, because children rely on adult caregivers who are also experiencing the direct effects of social risk factors, pediatric mental health must be understood in the context of familial and household relationships and the social needs of family members—the family unit is the patient.[30] In action, this translates to pediatric clinics partnering with adult-focused services and clinicians to work as a cohesive interdisciplinary team with caregivers and families, with the goal to improve the mental health of children.

Second, systemic racism deeply impacts and is entrenched within pediatric health care, mental health, and social health systems in the United States, creating inequity for families of color.[31–33] Pediatric clinicians and practices must apply an antiracist perspective and a strength-based approach as social and mental health care and service delivery pathways are introduced to avoid perpetuating existing structural inequities.[34–40] When possible, pediatric clinicians can also advocate for additional resources to promote the economic, social, and mental wellbeing of families and children.[36]

Antiracist and equitable strategies to support the social care and mental health of families includes.

- Highlight the strengths of parents and children in clinic notes, documentation, communication, and referrals that address social or mental health needs.

- Use language that recognizes that family functioning, social risks, and social needs stem from the structural Social Drivers of Health (SDOH) and not individual failure; for example, unreliable public transit as a cause of missed appointments rather than a mother failing to get a child to treatment.
- Prioritize parents' lived experiences by encouraging parents to identify the social and mental health needs that they would like support in addressing and acknowledging the needs identified by the family instead of what the clinician perceives as most important.
- Validate parents' perspectives regarding preferred intervention strategies to address identified concerns, being cognizant of clinician-client power imbalances.[41]
- Reflect cultural humility by expanding what clinicians perceive as "normal" or "standard" parenting behaviors to include the identities and values of the diverse parents and families served by the pediatric health care system.[41,42]

SUMMARY

The pediatric mental health crisis will demand that health care systems change what they do to better support children and adolescents and their families. Addressing and dismantling the systemic and structural barriers that have created pediatric mental health inequities will require also recognizing and intervening to mitigate the impacts of social inequities. Pediatric clinical teams can better integrate child mental and family social health to promote child well-being. Integrated care will maximize the likelihood of improving well-being across the lifespan.

CLINICS CARE POINTS

- During the ongoing youth mental health crisis, pediatric clinics can screen for both mental health and social health needs, linking to referrals guided by shared decision-making and family functioning principles, antiracist and culturally responsive practices.
- Pediatric clinicians can support families to understand the connections between mental health and social needs as well as the benefits of addressing them in tandem.
- Addressing mental health and social needs does not have to be the sole responsibility of the pediatric clinician but can be done collaboratively with social workers, behavioral health specialists, community health workers, community organizations, and health care payors.
- Addressing mental health and social needs in health care settings requires multi-sector partnerships to ensure key factors critical for success: (1) access to financial resources, (2) leveraging the power of various partners, and (3) equitable allocation of critical resources.

DISCLOSURES

The authors have no conflicts of interest relevant to this article to disclose.

FUNDING

Dr Anyigbo's effort on this work was supported by a career development award to the University of Cincinnati from the Center for Clinical and Translational Science and Training, UL1TR001425. Additional support for this work is derrived from the Administration for Health Research and Quality, R13HS028366 (PI: Gottlieb).

REFERENCES

1. AAP-AACAP-CHA Declaration of a National Emergency in Child and Adolescent Mental Health. Available at: https://www.aap.org/en/advocacy/child-and-adolescent-healthy-mental-development/aap-aacap-cha-declaration-of-a-national-emergency-in-child-and-adolescent-mental-health/?_ga=2.249322183.1932731054.1664157020-787450523.1647279228. [Accessed 25 September 2022].
2. Hyde R, O'Callaghan MJ, Bor W, et al. Long-term outcomes of infant behavioral dysregulation. Pediatrics 2012;130(5). https://doi.org/10.1542/peds.2010-3517.
3. 2022 National Healthcare Quality and Disparities Report. 2022. Available at: https://www.ncbi.nlm.nih.gov/books/NBK587174/. [Accessed 23 April 2024].
4. Kessler RC, Berglund P, Demler O, et al. Lifetime prevalence and age-of-onset distributions of DSM-IV disorders in the national comorbidity survey replication. Arch Gen Psychiatr 2005;62(6):593–602.
5. McGrath JJ, Al-Hamzawi A, Alonso J, et al. Age of onset and cumulative risk of mental disorders: a cross-national analysis of population surveys from 29 countries. Lancet Psychiatr 2023;10(9):668–81.
6. Copeland WE, Shanahan L, Costello EJ, et al. Childhood and adolescent psychiatric disorders as predictors of young adult disorders. Arch Gen Psychiatr 2009; 66(7):764–72.
7. Oerlemans AM, Wardenaar KJ, Raven D, et al. The association of developmental trajectories of adolescent mental health with early-adult functioning. PLoS One 2020;15(6). https://doi.org/10.1371/journal.pone.0233648.
8. Office of the Surgeon General (OSG). Protecting youth mental health. The U.S: Surgeon General's Advisory; 2021. Available at: https://www.ncbi.nlm.nih.gov/books/NBK575984/. [Accessed 23 April 2024].
9. Reiss F. Socioeconomic inequalities and mental health problems in children and adolescents: a systematic review. Soc Sci Med 2013;90:24–31.
10. Spencer AE, Baul TD, Sikov J, et al. The relationship between social risks and the mental health of school-age children in primary care. Acad Pediatr 2020;20(2): 208–15.
11. Johnson AD, Markowitz AJ. Food insecurity and family well-being outcomes among households with young children. J Pediatr 2018;196:275–82.
12. Anyigbo C, Liu C, Ehrlich S, et al. Household health-related social needs in newborns and infant behavioral functioning at 6 months. JAMA Pediatr 2023. https://doi.org/10.1001/jamapediatrics.2023.5721.
13. Vernon-Feagans L, Willoughby M, Garrett-Peters P, et al. Predictors of behavioral regulation in kindergarten: household chaos, parenting, and early executive functions. Dev Psychol 2016;52(3):430–41.
14. Klein RJ, Gyorda JA, Lekkas D, et al. Dysregulated emotion and trying substances in childhood: insights from a large nationally representative cohort study. Subst Use Misuse 2023;53(13):1625–33.
15. Petersen IT, Bates JE, Dodge KA, et al. Describing and predicting developmental profiles of externalizing problems from childhood to adulthood. Dev Psychopathol 2015;27(3):791–818.
16. Alegría M, Alvarez K, Cheng M, et al. Recent advances on social determinants of mental health: looking fast forward. Am J Psychiatr 2023;180(7):473–82.
17. Alegría M, NeMoyer A, Falgàs BI, et al. Social determinants of mental health: where we are and where we need to go. Curr Psychiatr Rep 2018;20(11). https://doi.org/10.1007/s11920-018-0969-9.

18. Hoffmann JA, Alegr ıa M, Alvarez K, et al. Disparities in pediatric mental and behavioral health conditions. Pediatrics 2022;150(4):2022058227. https://doi.org/10.1542/peds.2022-058227.
19. Cain KS, Meyer SC, Cummer E, et al. Association of food insecurity with mental health outcomes in parents and children. Acad Pediatr 2022;22(7):1105–14.
20. Mezzina R, Gopikumar V, Jenkins J, et al. Social vulnerability and mental health inequalities in the "syndemic": call for action. Front Psychiatry 2022;13:894370. https://doi.org/10.3389/fpsyt.2022.894370.
21. Kuhn J, Bair-Merritt M, Xuan Z, et al. Links between health-related social needs and mental health care disparities: implications for clinical practice clinical practice in pediatric psychology. Association 2020;2020(2):103–14.
22. Gottlieb LM, Hessler D, Wing H, et al. Revising the logic model behind health care's social care investments. Milbank Quarterly 2024. https://doi.org/10.1111/1468-0009.12690.
23. American Academy of Pediatrics. Screening Technical Assistance and Resource (STAR) Center. Available at: https://www.aap.org/en/patient-care/screening-technical-assistance-and-resource-center/. [Accessed 23 April 2024].
24. Shields-Zeeman L, Lewis C, Gottlieb L. Social and mental health care integration: the leading edge. JAMA Psychiatr 2019;76(9):881–2.
25. Castillo EG, Ijadi-Maghsoodi R, Shadravan S, et al. Community interventions to promote mental health and social equity. Curr Psychiatr Rep 2019;21(5):35.
26. Nelson KL. Associations between cross-sector partnerships and local health department participation in population-based activities to prevent mental health conditions. Am J Public Health 2020;110(S2):S225–31.
27. Liu PY, Beck AF, Lindau ST, et al. A framework for cross-sector partnerships to address childhood adversity and improve life course health. Pediatrics 2022; 149(Suppl 5):e2021053509O. https://doi.org/10.1542/peds.2021-053509O.
28. Kadakia KT, Offodile AC. The next generation of payment reforms for population health – An actionable agenda for 2035 informed by past gains and ongoing lessons. Milbank Quarterly 2023;101(S1):866–92.
29. Hoornbeek J, Chiyaka ET, Lanese B, et al. Financing community partnerships for health equity: findings and insights from cross-sector professionals. Health Serv Res 2024;59(S1). https://doi.org/10.1111/1475-6773.14237.
30. Lewandowski AS, Palermo TM, Stinson J, et al. Critical review systematic review of family functioning in families of children and adolescents with chronic pain. J Pain 2010;11(11):1027–38.
31. Braveman PA, Arkin E, Proctor D, et al. Systemic and structural racism: definitions, examples, health damages, and approaches to dismantling. Health Aff 2022;41(2):171–8.
32. Acker J, Aghaee S, Mujahid M, et al. Structural racism and adolescent mental health disparities in Northern California. JAMA Netw Open 2023;6(8):e2329825. https://doi.org/10.1001/jamanetworkopen.2023.29825.
33. Williams DT. Racism and the mechanisms maintaining racial stratification in Black families. J Family Theory 2023;15(2):206–18.
34. Heard-Garris NJ, Cale M, Camaj L, et al. Transmitting trauma: a systematic review of vicarious racism and child health. Soc Sci Med 2018;199:230–40.
35. Devaney C, Brady B, Crosse R, et al. Realizing the potential of a strengths-based approach in family support with young people and their parents. Child Fam Soc Work 2023;28(2):481–90.

36. DeNard C, Garcia A, Circo E. Caseworker perspectives on mental health disparities among racial/ethnic minority youth in child welfare. J Soc Serv Res 2017; 43(4):470–86.
37. Jain S, Reno R, Cohen AK, et al. Building a culturally-responsive, family-driven early childhood system of care: understanding the needs and strengths of ethnically diverse families of children with social-emotional and behavioral concerns. Child Youth Serv Rev 2019;100:31–8.
38. Williams A. Family support services delivered using a restorative approach: a framework for relationship and strengths-based whole-family practice. Child Fam Soc Work 2019;24(4):555–64.
39. Early T, GlenMaye L. Valuing families: social work practice with families from a strengths perspective. Soc Work 2000;45(2):118–30.
40. Yan Li AS, Lang Q, Cho J, et al. Cultural and structural humility and addressing systems of care disparities in mental health services for black, indigenous, and people of color youth. Child Adolesc Psychiatr Clin N Am 2022;31(2):251–9.
41. Gottlieb M. The case for a cultural humility framework in social work practice. J Ethn Cult Divers Soc Work 2021;30(6):463–81.
42. Ortega RM, Duntley-Matos R. Cultural sensitivity in the context of cultural humility. In: Encyclopedia of social work. 2020.

Innovative Approaches to Addressing Pediatric Mental Health

Digital Technologies in Pediatric Primary Care

Gary Maslow, MD, MPH[a,b,*], Richard Chung, MD[b],
Nicole Heilbron, PhD[b], Barbara Keith Walter, PhD, MPH[a]

KEYWORDS

• Mental health • Adolescent • Digital health

KEY POINTS

- There is a pediatric mental health crisis increasing rates of suicidal behavior among adolescents, with the greatest increase among adolescent girls that coincided with the coronavirus disease of 2019 (COVID-19) pandemic and may have accelerated the preexisting trend of worsening mental health for teens.
- Digital technologies can be used at multiple levels to support the mental health care of children including (1) health system/health care provider level; (2) patient–provider interface; (3) patient-facing consumer applications; and (4) new technology, including artificial intelligence.
- Health systems and health care providers have navigated a range of structural changes with the rapid expansion of the use of electronic health records over the past 2 decades, in addition to the rapid deployment of telehealth in the context of the COVID-19 pandemic.
- Collaborative Care Management is a structural approach to treating mental health conditions that was developed for mild/moderate depression.
- Apps that are specific to developmental screening have been created and can assist with the identification of common pediatric developmental conditions.

INTRODUCTION

Most mental health care for children starts in primary care. From developmental screening during early childhood to medication treatment of adolescent depression,

[a] Department of Psychiatry and Behavioral Sciences, Duke University School of Medicine, 2608 Erwin Road, Suite 300, Durham, NC 27705, USA; [b] Department of Pediatrics, Duke University School of Medicine, 3116 North Duke Street, Durham, NC 27705, USA
* Corresponding author. Department of Psychiatry and Behavioral Sciences, Duke University School of Medicine, 2068 Erwin Road, Suite 300, Durham, NC 27705.
E-mail address: gary.maslow@duke.edu

Pediatr Clin N Am 71 (2024) 1151–1164
https://doi.org/10.1016/j.pcl.2024.07.019 **pediatric.theclinics.com**
0031-3955/24/

children's mental health treatment is often connected to their primary care medical home. Pediatricians, family physicians, and advanced practice providers are asked to provide mental health care and yet many lack sufficient training opportunities. Digital technologies have been rapidly growing over the past decade that have the potential to support the care of pediatric patients. For both families and clinical providers, there remain many questions about how to judge these technologies and which tools can deliver on the promise of improved mental health through technology.

There is a pediatric mental health crisis with the centers for disease control and prevention (CDC) documenting increasing rates of suicidal behavior among adolescents, with the greatest increase among adolescent girls according to the most recent youth risk behavior surveillance system (YBRSS) report.[1] This increase coincided with the coronavirus disease of 2019 (COVID-19) pandemic and may have accelerated the pre-existing trend of worsening mental health for teens. The COVID-19 pandemic also resulted in the rapid adoption of telehealth as a form of mental health care that has persisted.[2]

Digital technologies can be used at multiple levels to support the mental health care of children including (1) health system/health care provider level; (2) patient–provider interface; (3) patient-facing consumer applications; and (4) new technology, including artificial intelligence (AI). At each of these levels, the novel technologies may lead to care improvements but also may have risks. One clear example is at the health system/health provider level. The use of electronic health records (EHRs) such as those widely deployed across the United States offer patients easy visibility into their health care records; however, these systems are also a primary source of physician burnout. Providers report spending more and more time documenting care and less time speaking directly with patients.

This article reviews the different digital technology interventions and provides primary care providers (PCPs) insight into this rapidly changing landscape.[3,4]

HEALTH SYSTEMS AND HEALTH CARE PROVIDER LEVEL APPLICATIONS IN DIRECT PATIENT CARE

Health systems and health care providers have navigated a range of structural changes with the rapid expansion of the use of EHRs over the past 2 decades, in addition to the rapid deployment of telehealth in the context of the COVID-19 pandemic.[5] These technological changes have had profound effects on the experience of providing pediatric care that are beyond the scope of this article. In examining innovative approaches to pediatric mental health care, it is important to acknowledge these 2 trends that are foundational to the current health care environment.

The EHR serves as a platform to link patients and providers and can allow providers to seek additional consultation easily. The EHR is a tool for deploying patient-facing questionnaires and to facilitate screening as discussed in the following section. The EHR also allows for the use of e-communications or e-consultation that allows a PCP to share a patient's chart with a consultant easily for review.[5] Providers are interested in this type of consultation, and with this type of additional support, they are able to provide care to children with mental health conditions.

Telehealth has grown, especially in the mental health field. The emergence of expanded coverage for telehealth assessment and treatment services during the COVID-19 pandemic accelerated a significant and widespread shift to the provision of mental health care via telehealth.[2] There are many different options for providing virtual care that are primary care based or that can be referral based. Although a comprehensive review of telehealth care in pediatric mental health is beyond the scope of this review, it is notable that primary care-based telehealth services can take various forms, including integrating mental health team members into the primary care visit without necessitating colocation. This provides opportunity for synchronous consultation and/or a virtual warm hand-off to the mental health team. Alternatively, a patient may be referred to behavioral health care via telehealth that is external to the primary care settings. In both cases, there is growing evidence that there are many potential benefits to the application of telehealth for direct patient care and consultation; however, there remains much to be learned about a range of considerations, including appropriateness and acceptability for particular types of services and work with specific populations of patients, and addressing disparities with respect to accessing care via telehealth.

One other innovative approach to primary care-based mental health care for children involves a model of care called "Collaborative Care Management" (CoCM). This approach is a structural approach to treating mental health conditions that was developed for mild/moderate depression. It fits within the category of digital innovations as it can be enhanced using a digital registry, as well as using text/telephone approaches to connecting with youth. CoCM for adult depression has over 70 randomized control trials supporting its efficacy. Recent studies have examined CoCM deployed for pediatric mental health conditions in primary care including attention deficit/hyperactivity disorder (ADHD), depression, and anxiety.[6–10] In this model, the PCP works with a behavioral health care manager (BHCM). The BHCM creates and maintains a registry of patients who have a specific behavioral health condition and monitors symptoms using evidence-based tools at regular intervals. The BHCM meets regularly with a child psychiatrist to review the registry and help make adjustments to the treatment plan. The BHCM communicates regularly through video, telephone, text, or in-person visits with a patient and their family and provides brief therapeutic interventions such as behavioral activation or parent coaching. Digital tools exist to support this model of care including from Advancing Integrated Mental Health Solutions Center at the University of Washington (AIMS) center that has a registry used across the country.[11]

PROVIDER-CONNECTED DIGITAL MENTAL HEALTH INTERVENTIONS: LINKING PROVIDERS TO PATIENTS AND PATIENTS TO INTERVENTIONS

Digital technologies can be deployed to support providers in caring for patients, as well as to link providers and patients through communication, and can be deployed as prescriptions that providers recommend to patients. Providers use patient-reported outcome measures and digital tracked screening tools regularly. Newer technologies including remote monitoring, mobile questionnaires, and wearable devices are becoming more widely available for a range of uses. Providers also have the ability to prescribe specific interventions that are evidence based including virtual reality, augmented reality programs, as well as novel computer games that have been studied as digital therapeutics.

As discussed earlier, the EHR is one of the most pervasive technologies that can be a part of addressing pediatric mental health. Particularly evidence-based screening approaches for children have been integrated into the EHR ranging from developmental screening in early childhood to mental health screening including depression screening in adolescents. The most simplistic version has been the incorporation of evidenced-based screeners, such as the Modified Checklist for Autism in Toddlers–Revised (M-CHAT-R/F) for autism, into the EHR in such a way that parents can directly provide answers to the questionnaire. There are many examples of this type of incorporation of screening into the EHR. In addition to just incorporating existing screening measures into the EHR platform, researchers have taken a further step in developing digital tools to enhance screening. One excellent example is the use of a digital phone-based app called "Sense to Know" that can be used by parents in conjunction with the M-CHAT-R/F to identify autism. This app involves video stimuli that children watch with their parents and the computer vision allows for assessment of markers of autism.[12,13] Combining the Sense to Know app with the M-CHAT-R/F increased the specificity of autism screening significantly.[13] Other types of apps that are specific to developmental screening have been created and can assist with the identification of common pediatric developmental conditions.

The use of the patient health questionnaire - 9 (PHQ-9) as a depression screen and tool for monitoring progress with depression treatment is another example of a screening approach where the digital connection between provider and patient can enhance care.[14,15] The PHQ-9 has been widely used as a screen and has been incorporated into the EHR broadly. There has also been the development of the collaborative care model for depression treatment that uses case managers as a part of the primary care team to improve depression outcomes through the use of a registry and monitoring the progress of adolescents with depression with regular biweekly symptom monitoring. This evidence-based model can be enhanced through the use of digital-based symptom monitoring. A care manager in partnership with a PCP can review the PHQ-9 with the patient and the data will be visible in the EHR allowing the PCP to more readily monitor progress. This type of symptom monitoring can be done using a care manager or through the use of apps as seen in monitoring other types of mental health symptoms. Suicidality and depression do not lend themselves as well to the use of remote monitoring as if there is a worsening of symptoms or presence of suicidality an immediate response is needed. ADHD is another condition for which the use of digital symptom monitoring can improve the quality of data that PCPs receive. The MeHealth portal was developed by researchers at Cincinnati Children's Hospital and provides a portal for PCPs to send and receive ADHD questionnaires with parents and teachers to modify ADHD treatment. This is one of several tools for this same purpose.

PATIENT/CONSUMER-FACING DIGITAL TECHNOLOGIES FOR PEDIATRIC MENTAL HEALTH

Mobile Mental Health Applications (mhealth Apps)

Over the past decade, there has also been a proliferation of consumer-facing mhealth apps that can be downloaded to smartphones or tablets to improve well-being, help patients set goals, track progress, or build in reminders, provide patient education, enhance diagnosis, connect to support or telehealth services, and improve symptom and treatment monitoring. The US Food and Drug Administration (FDA) released guidelines for regulating mhealth apps in 2015,[16,17] additional guidance has been evolving over the past 5 years, and there is now a Digital Center for Excellence at the FDA to address rapid changes and regulatory issues around digital health innovations.[18]

The release and download of mhealth apps to address anxiety, depression, and stress management significantly increased during the COVID-19 pandemic and over 90,000 digital apps were released in 2020 alone.[19] In addition, industry reports also suggest that the trend is projected to continue through the next several years. There are also many exciting private and public partnerships between academic centers and industry that are advancing innovation in mhealth.

Mental health apps are one type of mhealth apps and can be classified into several broad categories, with some of the most popular mental health apps listed in each category based on information from industry about users and downloads:

- Mindfulness, relaxation, and meditation apps to improve stress management and general well-being (Calm, Headspace, Insight Timer, 10% Happier, CosmicKids, Smiling Mind, and Breathe, Think, Do with Sesame)
- Mood and symptom tracking apps (Moodfit, Daylio, MoodTools)
- Cognitive behavioral therapy, dialectical behavior therapy, and/or self-help apps based on evidence-based therapies (Moodkit, Sanvello, Happify, MindShift CBT, DBT Coach, Calm Harm)
- Suicide prevention apps (Suicide Safe, Suicide Safety Plan, Virtual Hope Box, NotOK)
- Peer support apps (Talk life, Peer Collective, NotOK, MeeToo, and Hey Peers); some cognitive behavior therapy (CBT) apps like MindShift CBT also have a forum to provide or receive support from peers
- Mental health Chatbots that utilize AI (Wysa, Youper, Woebot)
- Telehealth apps to connect individuals with licensed professionals (BetterHelp, Talkspace, Talkiatry, Telehealth by Simple Practice, and Teen Counseling)
- Diagnosis-specific apps that include patient education and diagnosis, self-help, peer support, and/or telehealth (NOCD for obsessive complusive disorder [OCD], Recovery Record for eating disorders, PTSD Coach for post-traumatic stress disorder [PTSD])
- Gamified apps to improve mental health (Super Better, Sparx)

Apps often appeal to consumers because they are widely available, convenient, and accessible and meet a need at a time when there may be perceived barriers, including cost, stigma in seeking therapy, and a shortage of qualified mental health professionals. Industry data on how often mhealth apps are downloaded and individuals engage with them suggest that they are commonly used by adults.[20] However, concerns have been raised about consistent daily use of apps and the possible need to consider involving end users in development and gamifying apps to increase motivation and engagement so mhealth apps will not be abandoned.[21] Unfortunately, little information is available about how commonly mhealth apps are used by children and teens. However, available information from surveys about how teens engage with technology suggests that teens and young adults are using apps to improve general well-being and access peer support and increasingly researching information online and accessing blogs, podcasts, videos, and social media platforms for health information so it is important to know more about the potential benefits and risks.[22]

Increased demands for accessible apps as well as federal waivers on regulations during the COVID-19 Public Health Emergency also contributed to the expansion in development and use of digital health strategies. However, relatively few of those apps were rigorously studied with randomized controlled trials of their effectiveness. One company is also facing legal consequences of questionable business practices that influenced prescribing practices, did not protect private information, and made it difficult to cancel subscriptions that could erode public trust in digital health innovations.[23]

Direct-to-consumer mhealth and mobile mental health apps have the potential to reduce barriers, expand access to care, reduce disparities, enhance treatment, and improve self-management. Apps also have the potential to be used in conjunction with therapy and reinforce skills learned in therapy. They could also serve to be a useful first step in a stepped care, population health approach so that professionals can be available to deliver skilled interventions to the patients who need it the most as long as appropriate escalation pathways are in place, especially for youth at risk for suicide. However, many of these apps are still not well regulated, the quality of content is variable and sometimes not evidence-based, some are not effective or may be harmful, and some do not have appropriate protections in place for the privacy and security of the protected health information collected.[24] In addition, some of the apps have not included teens in development, been studied in teens, or included adequate representation of minority populations in clinical trials of effectiveness.[25,26]

There are also now so many mental health apps that models have been developed by the APA and Web sites have been developed to evaluate apps based on a variety of parameters such as cost, clinical focus, evidence, features, output, and privacy and security. App evaluations include Mind Apps (www.mindapps.org/) and One Mind Psyber Guide (https://onemindpsyberguide.org/) as detailed in excellent reviews.[19,27] In addition, some agencies such as the Veteran's Administration have also developed apps with evidence-based content to enhance treatment provided to patients and made the apps available to the patients as well as the general public to download for free, including COVID Coach, Mindfulness Coach, CBT-i Coach (for insomnia), PTSD Coach, and PTSD Family Coach. Some of these tools have also effectively been incorporated into patient care in "digital clinics" at the veterans administration (VA).[28]

Fortunately, as there has been exponential growth in mhealth apps, there have also been an increasing number of systematic reviews of effectiveness and there is support for effectiveness in the management of diabetes, hypertension, obesity, anxiety, and depression.[29,30] However, many questions remain about clinical effectiveness and strategies to integrate consumer-facing apps into treatment. Thus, it is clearly overwhelming for the average provider to keep up with rapidly changing digital health innovations and many questions remain about how helpful mhealth apps are for improving mental health and whether PCPs should recommend them to their patients. There is also little agreement between ratings and reviews on the app store, by professionals, and by the people who use the apps to help guide choices.[31] In addition, most patients are still less likely to use apps unless their provider recommends a specific app and research suggests that most individuals also experience difficulties with staying motivated to continue to use rather than abandon an app once it is downloaded.[32]

There is still much to learn about engaging youth in designing and consistently using evidence-based digital health tools.[33] Surveys and focus groups also suggest that individuals often identify apps through hearing about them from others, social media, or Internet searches rather than the recommendation of professionals.[34] In addition, although there are thousands of available apps to download, a relatively small number of apps are widely used and it has been recommended that PCPs consider a pragmatic approach to learning more about the most common apps, the way their patients use these apps, and the potential benefits and risks so they can provide informed guidance to their patients and emphasize that these digital health innovations are not meant to replace the advice of licensed professionals.[35]

Prescription Digital Therapeutics and Diagnostics

To respond to some of the criticism about mhealth apps, there was a significant increase in start-up companies to develop, test, and market evidence-based, innovative digital interventions, including prescription digital therapeutics that are regulated by the US FDA. Digital therapeutics are not the same as consumer-facing mhealth apps because they are evidence-based digital interventions to prevent, manage, or treat disorders that are regulated by the FDA and require a prescription. The FDA requires a rigorous review for approval. Some of the leaders in this industry have been Akili Interactive that developed EndeavorRx for pediatric ADHD (https://www.endeavorrx.com/) and Big Health (https://www.bighealth.com/), which developed Sleepio for insomnia (https://www.bighealth.com/sleepio/), Daylight for anxiety (https://www.bighealth.com/daylight/), and Spark Direct for depression (https://www.bighealth.com/spark-direct/). Some of these same companies are now revising their business strategy and also developing over the counter products that do not require a prescription because there has been a limited return on the substantial investment in developing these products even though there is a growing body of evidence that they may be beneficial.[36–38]

Another exciting innovation has been in the area of prescription diagnostics, including CanvasDx (https://cognoa.com/). CanvasDx uses an algorithm to analyze patterns in videos submitted by parents of behavior at home and questionnaires completed by a caregiver and a health care professional to determine if a child is likely to have autism spectrum disorder (ASD). It is meant to be used as an adjunct to the diagnostic evaluation by a trained professional and provides feedback within days rather than months that patients typically wait for an evaluation of possible autism and holds promise for earlier identification of at-risk children when used in conjunction with comprehensive diagnostic evaluations.

Some of the apps also integrate evidence-based diagnosis, treatment, and ongoing research to build the evidence base, such as the When to Wonder: Picky eating app and research study at NYU (https://nyulangone.org/news/child-psychiatrists-use-digital-technologies-advance- research-share-knowledge-enhance-access-care).

ARTIFICIAL INTELLIGENCE

As with many sectors, the advent of AI has been seen as potential transformative, disruptive, or dangerous for children with mental health conditions. The potential for expanding access to care is enormous and there are great concerns about privacy, algorithmic bias, and direct harm that may come from AI and AI-enabled mental health treatment. Examining the potential for AI is important and examining chatbots as a specific AI-powered intervention can help to illustrate the potential impact.

There are a wide array of potential applications of AI in pediatric mental health care, including in primary care. Significant positive impacts have already been observed in adult mental health care including improvements in diagnosis and treatment planning.[39,40] AI has also already demonstrated positive use cases in pediatric OCD,[41] ASD,[42] and ADHD.[43]

One key domain of application is improved diagnosis.[44,45] AI tools can access and synthesize a range of inputs including health records, online activities, and data from wearable devices to identify patterns suggestive of illness or distress and potentially predict behavioral health crises.[46,47] This is sometimes referred to as “personal sensing” or “digital phenotyping.” AI tools can assist human clinicians in synthesizing substantial amounts of information to optimize assessments and planning, and improve efficiency, and, consequently, access to care. In addition, natural language processing algorithms can detect patterns in textual content suggestive of distress or illness.[48] In addition, it may even be possible to use voice analysis to detect depression and anxiety among youth.[49]

Generative AI is able to provide novel content in response to user interactions, which may increase potential benefits but also broaden the potential risks, particularly if these tools are used by patients and families outside of a clinical relationship and clinical context. Large language models, such as ChatGPT, can be a helpful resource for pediatric mental health professionals and PCPs.[50] It can provide streamlined evidence-based guidance around assessment and management of common pediatric behavioral health issues. ChatGPT and similar resources may also be used by patients and families. In this way, it can be a complement to existing resources for both clinicians and families. The output of LLMs should be vetted appropriately and any content should be applied to the unique needs and circumstances of individual children and youth. Other ongoing efforts seek to use machine learning and AI to predict mental health trajectories among children and youth, potentially positioning clinicians to intervene far earlier than is currently possible.[51]

In general, applications of AI in mental health care have not been well studied among children and youth and substantial uncertainty and concern remain regarding the effectiveness, safety, and privacy of these resources and potential biases in underlying training datasets and algorithms. However, given these resources are readily accessible and not exclusively based on clinician recommendation or prescription, it is critical for clinicians to engage patients and families to understand if and how they are using these resources. Given the substantial uncertainties around AI applications in pediatric mental health care, PCPs should develop sufficient familiarity with these evolving resources to provide guidance to patients and families regarding both the potential benefits and risks of these tools.

Chatbots for Mental Health-Emerging Technology (Powered by Artificial Intelligence)

Chatbots have been incorporated into an array of use cases, including in health care. They have evolved overtime from rules-based chatbots linking keywords with automated responses to many current chatbots incorporating natural language processing algorithms and conversational AI to support effective engagement with user inputs that incorporate evidence-based mental health care techniques.[52–58] Most studies have focused on the use of chatbots in mental health care among adults. In a 2021 survey, 22% of adult respondents reported having used a mental health Chatbot, and among those, 44% used the Chatbot exclusively rather than seeking other care.[59]

In view of the ongoing mental health crisis among youth, there is substantial interest in using these tools in the care of youth.[60,61] Early studies in adolescents have suggested positive impacts on anxiety and depressive symptoms.[62] In one study of a Chatbot designed for youth with depression, 64.3% of participants indicated they would use the Chatbot in the future and 61.1% reported symptom improvement.[63] Another study demonstrated the feasibility, acceptability, usability, and safety of Chatbot-delivered CBT in youth with moderate depression presenting in primary care.[64] Another study of an AI-powered Chatbot used by college students with anxiety and depressive symptoms indicated usability and acceptability.[65] Further development to optimize engagement and outcomes will require continued engagement of youth themselves.[66]

Key benefits of chatbots include their constant availability and accessibility across populations, including in moments of acute crisis, without the structural barriers that typify traditional mental health services. Chatbots may also offer an avenue to care and support less riddled with a sense of stigma, judgment, or shame, given the absence of overt human engagement and the sense of privacy offered.[67,68] Given that many adolescents do not seek traditional mental health services and opt to cope with distressing symptoms alone,[69] chatbots may serve as an important entry point into care and support and could promote increased disclosure of mental health concerns. Chatbots may also have important applications in promoting resilience,[70] positive body image,[71] health behavior change, and treatment adherence[72] among youth.

Despite these potential benefits, notable questions remain regarding their usability, acceptability, effectiveness, privacy, safety, and potential for bias when used in pediatric mental health care.[73] As with other digital resources, concerns include overdependence on these outlets and supports at the expense of human interaction and care, increasing isolation, and concerns that digital resources are insufficient for severe, acute distress and may lead to unintended safety risks. In the pediatric primary care context, it is important for clinicians to be aware of these resources and tools and to inquire about their use among patients and families.

SUMMARY

Digital technologies, tools, and strategies have been a part of the health care landscape for the past 2 decades and have enhanced access to care, diagnosis, treatment, and communication between patients and health care teams. Digital tools have also been integrated into innovative models of evidence-based, patient-centered, population-based, and measurement-based care, such as CoCM. The growth in digital strategies for mental health has grown dramatically in the past few years with the significant expansion of telehealth during the COVID pandemic, increasing numbers of consumer-facing apps, digital mental health companies, and the acceleration of AI and nearly all national and international health organizations now have a digital health strategic plan. What this means for pediatric practices and providers caring for children is uncertain.[4] However, when combined with expertise from a qualified clinician, innovative digital technology tools hold tremendous promise for improving the quality of care and patient outcomes and reducing inequities, but they also hold risks that need to be recognized. This review aimed to provide an overview of the approaches to using digital tools to address mental health and support children and their families.[4]

CLINICS CARE POINTS

- EHR based tools can help with screening.
- Patients often use Apps and so asking about App use can be added to the patient interview related to mental health.
- There are many digital tools and looking to trusted source, such as the AAP to see if these tools are evidence based is important.

DISCLOSURE

The authors have nothing to disclose. Also, this article was not suppored by any research funding.

REFERENCES

1. Centers for Disease Control and Prevention. Youth risk behavior surveillance system (YRBSS) 2023. Available at: https://www.cdc.gov/healthyyouth/data/yrbs/questionnaires.htm. [Accessed 1 May 2024].

2. Cunningham NR, Ely SL, Barber Garcia BN, et al. Addressing pediatric mental health using telehealth during Coronavirus Disease-2019 and beyond: A narrative review. Acad Pediatr 2021;21(7):1108–17.
3. Bouabida K, Lebouché B, Pomey MP. Telehealth and COVID-19 Pandemic: An overview of the telehealth use, advantages, challenges, and opportunities during COVID-19 pandemic. Healthcare (Basel) 2022;10(11):2293. PMID: 36421617; PMCID: PMC9690761.
4. Insel T. Digital mental health care: five lessons from Act 1 and a preview of Acts 2–5. NPJ Digit. Med 2023;6:9.
5. Rai M, Vigod SN, Hensel JM. Barriers to office-based mental health care and interest in e-communication with providers: A survey study. JMIR Ment Health 2016; 3(3):e35. Published 2016 Aug 1.
6. Kolko DJ, Campo J, Kilbourne AM, et al. Collaborative care outcomes for pediatric behavioral health problems: a cluster randomized trial. Pediatrics 2014;133(4): e981–92.
7. Campo JV, Geist R, Kolko DJ. Integration of pediatric behavioral health services in primary care: Improving access and outcomes with collaborative care. Can J Psychiatr 2018;63(7):432–8.
8. Silverstein M, Hironaka LK, Walter HJ, et al. Collaborative care for children with ADHD symptoms: a randomized comparative effectiveness trial. Pediatrics 2015;135(4):e858–67.
9. Kodish I, Richardson L, Schlesinger A. Collaborative and integrated care for adolescent depression. Child Adolesc Psychiatr Clin N Am 2019;28(3):315–25.
10. Richardson LP, Ludman E, McCauley E, et al. Collaborative care for adolescents with depression in primary care: a randomized clinical trial. JAMA 2014;312(8): 809–16.
11. Aims Center, University of Washington. Registries for Collaborative Care. 2023. Aims Center. Available at: https://aims.uw.edu/. [Accessed 10 May 2024].
12. Coffman M, Di Martino JM, Aiello R, et al. Relationship between quantitative digital behavioral features and clinical profiles in young autistic children. Autism Res 2023;16(7):1360–74.
13. Perochon S, Di Martino JM, Carpenter KLH, et al. Early detection of autism using digital behavioral phenotyping. Nat Med 2023;29(10):2489–97.
14. McCue M, Blair C, Fehnert B, et al. Mobile App to Enhance Patient Activation and Patient-Provider Communication in Major Depressive Disorder Management: Collaborative, Randomized Controlled Pilot Study. JMIR Form Res 2022;6(10): e34923. https://doi.org/10.2196/34923. Published 2022 Oct 27.
15. Nickels S, Edwards MD, Poole SF, et al. Toward a Mobile Platform for Real-world Digital Measurement of Depression: User-Centered Design, Data Quality, and Behavioral and Clinical Modeling. JMIR Ment Health 2021;8(8):e27589. https://doi.org/10.2196/27589. Published 2021 Aug 10.
16. Mehealth for ADHD. Cincinatti Children's Hospital Medical Center. Available at: https://www.mehealth.com/. [Accessed 10 June 2024].
17. Food and Drug Administration. Mobile Medical Applications: Guidance for Industry and Food and Drug Administration Staff. 2015. Available at: https://www.fda.gov/media/80958/download.
18. Watson A, Chapman R, Shafai G, et al. FDA regulations and prescription digital therapeutics: Evolving with the technologies they regulate. Front Digit Health 2023;5:1086219. https://doi.org/10.3389/fdgth.2023.1086219. PMID: 37139487; PMCID: PMC10150093.

19. Lagan S, Aquino P, Emerson MR, et al. Actionable health app evaluation: translating expert frameworks into objective metrics. NPJ Digit Med 2020;3:100.
20. Paradis S, Roussel J, Bosson JL, et al. Use of smartphone health apps among patients aged 18 to 69 years in primary care: Population-based cross-sectional survey. JMIR Form Res 2022;6(6):e34882. https://doi.org/10.2196/34882. PMID: 35708744; PMCID: PMC9247815.
21. Mustafa AS, Ali N, Dhillon JS, et al. User engagement and abandonment of mHealth: A cross-sectional survey. Healthcare 2022;10:221.
22. Rideout V. Fox, susannah; and well being trust, "digital health practices, social media use, and mental well-being among teens and young adults in the U.S. Articles; 2018. p. 1093. *Abstracts, and Reports.*
23. Office of the NY State Attorney General Leticia James Attorney General James Secures $740,000 from Online Mental Health Provider for its Burdensome Cancellation Process. Press Release. Available at: https://ag.ny.gov/press-release/2023/attorney-general-james-secures-740000-online-mental-health-provider-its. [Accessed 10 May 2024].
24. Akbar S, Coiera E, Magrabi F. Safety concerns with consumer-facing mobile health applications and their consequences: a scoping review. J Am Med Inform Assoc 2020;27(2):330–40. PMID: 31599936; PMCID: PMC7025360.
25. McGorry PD, Mei C, Chanen A, et al. Designing and scaling up integrated youth mental health care. World Psychiatr 2022;21(1):61–76. PMID: 35015367; PMCID: PMC8751571.
26. Adu-Brimpong J, Pugh J, Darko D, et al. Examining diversity in digital therapeutics clinical trials: Descriptive analysis. J Med Internet Res 2023;25:e37447 (APA reference–.
27. Ribaut J, DeVito Dabbs A, Dobbels F, et al. Developing a comprehensive list of criteria to evaluate the characteristics and quality of eHealth smartphone apps: Systematic review. JMIR Mhealth Uhealth 2024;12:e48625. https://doi.org/10.2196/48625. Available at: https://mhealth.jmir.org/2024/1/e48625.
28. Connolly SL, Kuhn E, Possemato K, et al. Digital clinics and mobile technology implementation for mental health care. Curr Psychiatry Rep 2021;23(7):38. PMID: 33961135; PMCID: PMC8103883.
29. Chong SOK, Pedron S, Abdelmalak N, et al. An umbrella review of effectiveness and efficacy trials for app-based health interventions. NPJ Digit. Med 2023;6:233.
30. Wright M, Reitegger F, Cela H, et al. Interventions with digital tools for mental health promotion among 11-18 Year Olds: A systematic review and meta-Analysis. J Youth Adolesc 2023;52(4):754–79. Epub 2023 Feb 8. PMID: 36754917; PMCID: PMC9907880.
31. Hudson G, Negbenose E, Neary M, et al. Comparing professional and consumer ratings of mental health apps: Mixed methods study. JMIR Form Res 2022;6(9):e39813. https://doi.org/10.2196/39813. PMID: 36149733; PMCID: PMC9547331.
32. Mustafa AS, Ali N, Dhillon JS, et al. User engagement and abandonment of mHealth: A cross-sectional survey. Healthcare 2022;10:221, healthcare10020221.
33. Liverpool S, Mota C, Sales C, et al. Engaging children and young people in digital mental health interventions: Systematic review of modes of delivery, facilitators, and barriers. J Med Internet Res 2020;22(6):e16317. https://doi.org/10.2196/16317.
34. Schueller S, Neary M, O'Loughlin K, et al. Discovery of and interest in health Apps Among Those With Mental Health Needs: Survey and Focus Group Study. J Med Internet Res 2018;20(6):e10141. https://doi.org/10.2196/10141. Available at: https://www.jmir.org/2018/6/e10141.

35. Schueller SM, Wasil AR, Bunyi J, et al. Mental health apps for children and adolescents: A clinician-friendly review. J Am Acad Child Adolesc Psychiatry 2024; 63(4):389–92.e1.
36. Davis NO, Bower J, Kollins SH. Proof-of-concept study of an at-home, engaging, digital intervention for pediatric ADHD. PLoS One 2018;13(1):e0189749. https://doi.org/10.1371/journal.pone.0189749. PMID: 29324745; PMCID: PMC5764249.
37. Kollins SH, Childress A, Heusser AC, et al. Effectiveness of a digital therapeutic as adjunct to treatment with medication in pediatric ADHD. npj Digit. Med 2021; 4:58.
38. Evans SW, Beauchaine TP, Chronis-Tuscano A, et al. The efficacy of cognitive videogame training for ADHD and what FDA clearance means for clinicians. Evidence-Based Practice in Child and Adolescent Mental Health 2021;6(1):116–30.
39. Bateman K. 4 ways artificial intelligence is improving mental health therapy. World Economic Forum; 2021. Available at: https://www.weforum.org/agenda/2021/12/ai-mental-health-cbt-therapy/. [Accessed 19 March 2024].
40. Rapid growth in AI mental health technology prompts optimism and concerns. RTI Health Advance; 2023. Available at: https://healthcare.rti.org/insights/ai-mental-health-technology. [Accessed 19 March 2024].
41. Lenhard F, Sauer S, Andersson E, et al. Prediction of outcome in internet-delivered cognitive behaviour therapy for paediatric obsessive-compulsive disorder: A machine learning approach. Int J Methods Psychiatr Res 2018;27(1): e1576. https://doi.org/10.1002/mpr.1576.
42. Wall DP, Dally R, Luyster R, et al. Use of artificial intelligence to shorten the behavioral diagnosis of autism. PLoS One 2012;7(8):e43855. https://doi.org/10.1371/journal.pone.0043855.
43. Rahman MM. AI for ADHD: Opportunities and challenges. J Atten Disord 2023; 27(8):797–9.
44. Vial T, Almon A. Artificial intelligence in mental health therapy for children and adolescents. JAMA Pediatr 2023;177(12):1251–2.
45. D'Alfonso S. AI in mental health. Current Opinion in Psychology 2020;36:112–7.
46. Walsh CG, Ribeiro JD, Franklin JC. Predicting risk of suicide attempts over time through machine learning. Clin Psychol Sci 2017;5(3):457–69.
47. Garriga R, Mas J, Abraha S, et al. Machine learning model to predict mental health crises from electronic health records. Nat Med 2022;28(6):1240–8.
48. Zhang T, Schoene AM, Ji S, et al. Natural language processing applied to mental illness detection: a narrative review. NPJ Digit Med 2022;5(1):46. Published 2022 Apr 8.
49. McGinnis EW, Anderau SP, Hruschak J, et al. Giving Voice to Vulnerable Children: Machine Learning Analysis of Speech Detects Anxiety and Depression in Early Childhood. IEEE J Biomed Health Inform 2019;23(6):2294–301.
50. van Schalkwyk G. Artificial intelligence in pediatric behavioral health. Child Adolesc Psychiatry Ment Health 2023;17(1):38. PMID: 36907862; PMCID: PMC10009954.
51. Nature Research Custom Media. Cincinnati Children's. Scientists, Supercomputers and AI Seek to Decode Childhood Mental Health. Nature Portfolio. Available at: https://www.nature.com/articles/d42473-022-00339-z. [Accessed 19 March 2024].
52. Fitzpatrick KK, Darcy A, Vierhile M. Delivering cognitive behavior therapy to young adults with symptoms of depression and anxiety Using a Fully Automated Conversational Agent (Woebot): A Randomized Controlled Trial. JMIR Ment Health 2017;4(2):e19. https://doi.org/10.2196/mental.7785. Published 2017 Jun 6.

53. Inkster B, Sarda S, Subramanian V. An empathy-driven, conversational Artificial Intelligence agent (Wysa) for digital mental well-being: Real-world data evaluation mixed-methods study. JMIR Mhealth Uhealth 2018;6(11):e12106. https://doi.org/10.2196/12106. Published 2018 Nov 23.
54. Gordon C Replika. Launches New Immersive AI Wellness Avatar Experience. Forbes. Available at: https://www.forbes.com/sites/cindygordon/2024/01/30/replika-launches-new-immersive-ai-wellness-avatar-experience/?sh=7ddab9ea1fe2. [Accessed 19 March 2024].
55. Ta V, Griffith C, Boatfield C, et al. User experiences of social support from companion chatbots in everyday contexts: Thematic analysis. J Med Internet Res 2020;22(3):e16235. https://doi.org/10.2196/16235. Published 2020 Mar 6.
56. Mehta A, Niles AN, Vargas JH, et al. Acceptability and effectiveness of artificial intelligence therapy for anxiety and depression (Youper): Longitudinal observational study. J Med Internet Res 2021;23(6):e26771. https://doi.org/10.2196/26771. Published 2021 Jun 22.
57. Fulmer R, Joerin A, Gentile B, et al. Using psychological artificial intelligence (Tess) to relieve symptoms of depression and anxiety: Randomized controlled trial. JMIR Ment Health 2018;5(4):e64. https://doi.org/10.2196/mental.9782. Published 2018 Dec 13.
58. Abd-Alrazaq AA, Alajlani M, Alalwan AA, et al. An overview of the features of chatbots in mental health: A scoping review. Int J Med Inform 2019;132:103978. https://doi.org/10.1016/j.ijmedinf.2019.103978.
59. Martinengo L, Lum E, Car J. Evaluation of chatbot-delivered interventions for self-management of depression: Content analysis. J Affect Disord 2022;319:598–607.
60. Opel DJ, Kious BM, Cohen IG. AI as a mental health therapist for adolescents. JAMA Pediatr 2023;177(12):1253–4.
61. Andrew J, Rudra M, Eunice J, et al. Artificial intelligence in adolescents mental health disorder diagnosis, prognosis, and treatment. Front Public Health 2023;11:1110088. https://doi.org/10.3389/fpubh.2023.1110088. Published 2023 Mar 31.
62. Lim SM, Shiau CWC, Cheng LJ, et al. Chatbot-delivered psychotherapy for adults with depressive and anxiety symptoms: A systematic review and meta-regression. Behav Ther 2022;53(2):334–47.
63. Dosovitsky G, Bunge E. Development of a chatbot for depression: adolescent perceptions and recommendations. Child Adolesc Ment Health 2023;28(1):124–7.
64. Nicol G, Wang R, Graham S, et al. Chatbot-delivered cognitive behavioral therapy in adolescents with depression and anxiety during the COVID-19 pandemic: Feasibility and acceptability study. JMIR Form Res 2022;6(11):e40242. https://doi.org/10.2196/40242. Published 2022 Nov 22.
65. Klos MC, Escoredo M, Joerin A, et al. Artificial intelligence-based chatbot for anxiety and depression in university students: Pilot randomized controlled trial. JMIR Form Res 2021;5(8):e20678. https://doi.org/10.2196/20678. Published 2021 Aug 12.
66. Thai K, Tsiandoulas KH, Stephenson EA, et al. Perspectives of youths on the ethical use of artificial intelligence in health care research and clinical care. JAMA Netw Open 2023;6(5):e2310659. https://doi.org/10.1001/jamanetworkopen.2023.10659. Published 2023 May 1.
67. Haque MDR, Rubya S. An overview of chatbot-based mobile mental health apps: Insights from app description and user reviews. JMIR Mhealth Uhealth 2023;11:e44838. https://doi.org/10.2196/44838. Published 2023 May 22.

68. Lee Y, Yamashita N, Huang Y. Designing a chatbot as a mediator for promoting deep self-disclosure to a real mental health professional. Proc. ACM Hum.-Comput 2020;4:CSCW1.
69. Radez J, Reardon T, Creswell C, et al. Why do children and adolescents (not) seek and access professional help for their mental health problems? A systematic review of quantitative and qualitative studies. Eur Child Adolesc Psychiatry 2021;30(2):183–211.
70. Holt-Quick C, Warren J, Stasiak K, et al. A chatbot architecture for promoting youth resilience. Healthier Lives, Digitally Enabled 2021;99–105. https://doi.org/10.3233/shti210017.
71. Beilharz F, Sukunesan S, Rossell SL, et al. Development of a positive body image chatbot (KIT) with young people and parents/carers: Qualitative focus group study. J Med Internet Res 2021;23(6):e27807. https://doi.org/10.2196/27807. Published 2021 Jun 16.
72. Zhang J, Oh YJ, Lange P, et al. Artificial intelligence chatbot behavior change model for designing artificial intelligence chatbots to promote physical activity and a healthy diet: Viewpoint. J Med Internet Res 2020;22(9):e22845. https://doi.org/10.2196/22845. Published 2020 Sep 30.
73. Kretzschmar K, Tyroll H, Pavarini G, et al, NeurOx Young People's Advisory Group. Can your phone be your therapist? young people's ethical perspectives on the use of fully automated conversational agents (chatbots) in mental health support. Biomed Inform Insights 2019;11:1178222619829083.

A "Next Generation" of Pediatric Mental Health Systems

Lawrence S. Wissow, MD, MPH[a,*], Laura P. Richardson, MD, MPH[b,1]

KEYWORDS

• Children's mental health • Prevention • Primary care • Social determinants of health

KEY POINTS

- The context of children's mental health care is rapidly changing because of global demographic, socio-economic, and climatic shifts.
- Changes in health care financing and challenges to support for universal public education could pose opportunities or further challenges for mental health services.
- Next generation services will need full integration of services that address social determinants of health (including caregivers' mental health needs).
- New approaches to screening, transdiagnostic treatment, and predicting responsiveness to initial treatment will replace current screening and stepped care models.
- The next generation of services will be composed of novel screening and treatment methods embedded in "rediscovered" models of care that center relationships, comprehensiveness, and responsiveness to communities.

INTRODUCTION

Newspaper columnist Mary Schmich once wrote a list of important facts for young people (often mis-attributed to a graduation speech by the author Kurt Vonnegut).[1] Chief among her facts was that one should not worry about the future, because, she said, "the real troubles in your life are apt to be things that never crossed your worried mind, the kind that blindside you at 4 PM on some idle Tuesday."

Trying to predict the future based on any present state is similarly fraught. We really do not know what transformative development (think CRISPR) might appear out of an obscure (to us, at least) corner of science and change everything. So it is with describing a next generation of mental health systems serving children, youth, and

[a] Division of Child and Adolescent Psychiatry, Department of Psychiatry and Behavioral Sciences, School of Medicine, University of Washington, Seattle, WA, USA; [b] Department of Pediatrics, School of Medicine, University of Washington, Seattle, WA, USA
[1] Present address: 4540 Sand Point Way, Suite 200, Seattle WA 98105.
* Corresponding author. Department of Psychiatry, Box 356560, Seattle, WA 98195-7238.
E-mail address: lwissow@uw.edu

Pediatr Clin N Am 71 (2024) 1165–1182
https://doi.org/10.1016/j.pcl.2024.07.020 pediatric.theclinics.com

their families. It is relatively easy to describe likely challenges, and to say what works and does not in our present system. It is a lot harder to predict what a future system will look like. In that spirit, this article aims first to set out some observations about how the context of child, youth, and family mental health care is shifting, some limitations of the current system, and principles that could drive the structure and function of a future system. In putting these ideas forward, the authors of this article acknowledge the many ideas they have learned from colleagues and the fact that we write largely from the perspective of clinicians and researchers.

CHANGING CHILD, YOUTH, AND FAMILY CONTEXT

Several forces are changing the context in which child, youth, and family mental health services need to be delivered. Some impact the incidence and treatability of mental health problems; some change the populations coming to treatment, and others challenge the fundamental person-to-person nature of treatment that underlies present ideals.[2]

One of the strongest forces changing the context for child and youth mental health services is the migration and displacement of children and their families. In 2020, the number of people globally who were forced from their homes because of human or natural disasters reached its highest recorded level of 89.4 million.[3] While overall children and youth make up about 30% of the world population, they make up about 41% of the world population of refugees.[4] Children living outside their country of birth are much more likely to be refugees than are adults, and refugee children have higher rates of mental health problems compared to peers, especially when they arrive unaccompanied.[5]

A related aspect of context is the global trend toward increasing socioeconomic disparities. In the United States (US), the concentration of wealth among the wealthiest families continues to increase, as do the gaps between the assets of white versus Black and Hispanic families and between older versus younger families.[6] These wealth gaps are mirrored in access to health care and in health outcomes.[7] Gaps related to inequalities are seen even in countries with universal health care. A study in Germany[8] found that children and youth living in lower income households had a higher risk of developing mental health problems, even when accounting for the higher levels of stress associated with low income. We know that both absolute and relative poverty are associated with negative developmental, health and mental health outcomes.[9] Socio-economic status, for example, strongly influences children's cognitive development over the first decade of life, independently of their cognitive development in infancy, and early life. Conversely, programs that target key impacts of poverty and income disparities demonstrate the potential to improve cognitive functions such as implicit learning, inhibitory control (a key component of attention), and long-term memory that are essential to later learning and emotional health.[10]

Climate change is also having an impact on children's well-being and will likely have more. Its impact can be both direct, in causing changes to the environment that impact infectious disease, nutrition, family resources, or disruptions to community services, or indirectly through forced or voluntary relocation of families within countries or abroad.[11] The children of women who experience extreme climate events during pregnancy, and children who live through these events in the first years of their lives, demonstrate negative impacts to their cognitive development.[12,13]

Another area of contextual change—or at least uncertainty—is what will become of public education in the US and globally. Education has been recognized internationally as a basic human right. School readinesses, and academic and social success in school, are strong determinants of children's positive mental health, resilience, and long-term social and economic success.[14] However, there remain challenges to financing universal public education, as well as challenges to its inclusivity, to the nature (and control over) of its content, and its extension to early childhood.[15] Globally, UNESCO estimates that 58% of children and adolescents worldwide have not reached minimal proficiency levels in language and math. Though the percentage is lowest in Europe and North America, these attainment gaps are still 17% for males and 12% for females in those regions.[16] The current US federal government has outlined a multi-faceted plan to reduce inequalities in access to basic and higher education, including stabilizing and enhancing the resources supporting education for historically under-served communities, but the extent to which these policies will succeed or be sustained is not known.[17]

And while one could list many other contextual changes, the impact of technology stands out as both a threat and promise (**Table 1**). Rapid changes to service delivery during the coronavirus pandemic brought tele-mental health services from a relatively little used tool to a mainstay of service delivery. Other digital tools offer the possibility of reducing the burden of note writing, tailoring follow-up protocols to make them more effective and efficient, and making self-guided treatment more widely available and better tailored to individual needs (including adaptations in multiple languages and for varying levels of literacy). However, the impact of these innovations remains

Table 1
Contextual challenges and future responses

Forces Driving Change	Design of a Future System
Context and populations	
• Internal and external migration (including refugees) driving cultural diversity • Increasing socio-economic disparities • Climate change as a source of stress and driver of migration • Challenges to the availability of universal public education • Impact of technology on standards for delivery of "interpersonal" services	• Systematic planning systems at local level based on family and youth input • Cross-sector planning to build or sustain health promoting communities • Further integration of mental health into community social programs, early childhood education, and schools • Modeling use of tele- vs in-person services to provide maximal access without sacrificing personal contact • Coached use of on-line self-help materials
Financing uncertainty and persistent barriers	
• Uneven, fee-for-service system recognized as distorting care away from evidence-based early intervention and non-acute services • Consolidation of ownership threatens interpersonal aspects of care and pushes mental health care toward medical models • Inability to fully integrate attention to social determinants perpetuates medicalizing problems with predominantly social or economic "treatments" • Inability of child-focused systems to effectively offer treatment to parents	• Shift of base of community mental health to primary care for focus on universal access, prevention, early treatment • Return to models for primary care that have human scale and flexibility • Full integration of attention to social determinants within primary care; social determinants have equal place in differential diagnosis and treatment planning • Through changes to regulations, training, and staffing child-focused clinical sites develop capacity to address parental mental health problems

uncertain. Studies to date do not yet give a clear picture of when tele-delivered treatment is acceptable and when it is not, and there are concerns that it may increase disparities in service access.[18]

Digital self-help tools have strong evidence of effectiveness, but they appear to work best when used in the context of human coaching.[19] One of their most exciting potentials is that they could be a piece of scalable interventions that can be provided to individuals who currently are screened out of services as not yet meeting diagnostic thresholds.[20,21] Online prevention interventions have shown the ability to improve quality-of-life and reduce symptoms among individuals who experience impairment but who might not otherwise qualify for treatment. These tools can combine a variety of forms of treatment and offer the potential of being deployed by primary care, schools, or other community sites where young people may reveal that they have early indications of mood problems. On-line preventive interventions may also address the problem that by the time many youth come for mental health care they already are experiencing considerable morbidity,[22] making their conditions harder to treat. In Australia, Project Synergy has been an attempt to create an on-line entry point for mental health services whose goal was not to replace the face to face system but rather to augment it with more effective screening, including assessment of strengths, and connect young people to the most appropriate services for prevention or treatment.[23]

UNCERTAINTY ABOUT HOW CARE WILL BE FINANCED IN THE FUTURE

We also do not know what the future of health care financing is in the US (where universal coverage remains a goal) and countries like the United Kingdom (UK) (where universal coverage is being challenged) and in many lower income countries where only basic health services remain available without out-of-reach personal expenditures. In the US, the fee for service system constitutes a major barrier to accessing mental health care for children and youth.[24] Access through public sector payers and services is limited by an ongoing lack of parity between payment for mental health services and other medical services. Underfunded public services also suffer from high rates of clinician turnover and low uptake of evidence-based services.[25,26] Access for families with commercial insurance is limited by the fact that many community-based mental health providers function only on a cash basis, charging fees that are only partly reimbursed by insurers, if at all. Health care spending (or limits on parents' ability to work if their children have significant developmental, behavioral, or emotional problems) can drive families into poverty.[27] Within international agencies, there is a consensus that basic universal health care access is a necessary step toward achieving development goals. Many countries including the US are still far from providing universal access and progress has slowed, with ongoing disparities in child and maternal services versus access to services for adults.

An important artifact of the way mental health care is financed is the predominance of time-limited treatment for what can be chronic conditions. There are many good reasons to develop short-term therapies, even those that have the potential to be delivered in a single session.[28] Individuals often seek help at a time of crisis, and help in that moment can restore a situation to equilibrium. In addition, many time-limited psychologic treatments are designed to teach skills or create new patterns of behavior that can be sustained after the treatment ends. But because mental health treatment resources are so severely limited relative to the prevalence of conditions, time-limited treatment also serves the purpose of clearing space for the next patient on the waiting list. This might work well if mental health treatment was definitive, like taking out an inflamed appendix. However, many mental health conditions recur either at times of stress, developmental transitions, or out of the blue, and while many patients are demonstrably better at the end of their time-limited treatment, many are not symptom free. Increasingly, primary care practices have registries and mechanisms to track and monitor patients with chronic problems, trying to identify the risk of relapse before it occurs, but this is not a common practice in mental health care.[29]

Another financing unknown is the consolidation of ownership of medical facilities and practices by large entities that are explicitly or function similarly to profit-making corporations.[30,31] Though in some cases consolidation can bring stability to some smaller, often rural sites of care, overall they have a history of driving up the price of services and, perhaps most importantly for mental health care, reducing flexibility and continuity, which are essential aspects of care for engaging families in care and providing services that meet family needs.[32] The loss of continuity and the increasing distribution of care functions to call or scheduling centers is particularly of concern, given the importance of relationships and therapeutic alliance to many aspects of mental health care ranging from willingness to disclose concerns to building an effective relationship with clinicians.[33] Large organizations of necessity rely heavily on "standard work" and frequently on out-sourcing or consolidating key functions ranging from scheduling patients to managing relationships with clinical staff. These approaches may work well in some very highly technical and necessarily standardized aspects of medical care—notably surgery and intensive care—but fail to recognize the very different nature of work in primary care and mental health, where engaging patients around their unique and constantly evolving needs is what is "standard."[34]

Finally, some questions about financing reflect the recognition that the "biopsychosocial" model of health is poorly reflected in the separation of medical and social expenditures. In some countries, there are experiments with providing municipalities with global funding for youth wellness that the cities can allocate as they wish to physical health, mental health, social needs, and other community programs including both preventive and indicated care.[35–37] Finance is often the driving force behind these efforts—they target increasing global costs—and as such they have the potential to squeeze services. But they also offer the opportunity to correct the imbalance of expenditures and effort between preventive/early intervention services and more specialized treatment. In the Netherlands, an approach to this global model has been to split out child and youth preventive services from "curative" services (which are financed separately).[38] Specialized teams that include generalist physicians with extra mental health training systematically engage families in preventive care and have access to a wide range of social and educational resources. The long-term impact of this approach remains to be seen; in the short-term, in the Netherlands, it may not have reduced the need for specialized child/youth mental health services, but it has been projected to have a strong positive return on investment over the lifespan.

In the US, the Center for Medicare and Medicaid Innovation launched the Integrated Care for Kids (InCK) trials in 7 communities targeting early identification of psychosocial problems, stratifying services by risk, and collaboration across community services.[39] In the North Carolina InCK program,[40] screening in primary care plus the aggregation of the data from Medicaid, juvenile justice, and social services systems identify levels of risk that qualify families for different levels of services (including a centralized care management program) and practices for different levels of payment. Part of the effort to have a broad focus on early childhood is a "kindergarten readiness bundle" that includes both universal and indicated supports for families with young children. Practices will be able to receive supplemental payments for implementing the bundle; the program will monitor, but not hold practices responsible for, actual readiness assessments of InCK-enrolled children as they enter school.

Of course, the elephant in the social determinants room for pediatricians, child psychiatrists, psychologists, and other clinicians who practice in systems built around these child-serving professions, is that parents and family are the primary "social determinant" in children's lives. Pediatrics in particular has based the justification for its specialty on the premise that "children are not little adults." While this is clearly true and critical to the proper medical care of children, it has in many countries, including the US, created a system in which children and their parents cannot receive coordinated treatment for conditions where there is a demonstrable 2-way relationship between the welfare of the child and parent. To take only 1 example, meta-analyses find that treating parental depression improves child mental health, and treating children improves parental mental health.[41,42] Yet outside of screening for maternal depression in the post-partum period, pediatricians do not have the capacity to address parental mood or substance problems, and most child mental health service systems do not offer coordinated care for children and their families. A 2017 report from the US Substance Abuse and Mental Health Services Administration (SAMSHA) estimated that over 12% of US children under 18 (about 8.7 million children) lived with a parent who had a substance use disorder.[43] Children living in families where parents have these disorders experience a number of direct and indirect impacts on their health and development, many of which cannot be adequately treated while the parent's disorder goes untreated.[44]

LIMITS OF CURRENT APPROACHES TO SCREENING, DIAGNOSIS, AND TREATMENT

The concept of screening—systematically searching for individuals who might be connected with care—is at the core of population-based approaches to reducing the burden of mental health problems. Simple instruments such as the Strengths and Difficulties Questionnaire, Pediatric Symptom Checklist, and Patient Health Questionnaire have had a transformative impact on institutionalizing mental health as part of general medical care, but as clinical tools they pose a number of problems including low positive predictive values and the need for additional stages of screening.[45] Newer approaches may combine brief questionnaires with the ability of artificial intelligence to assess either video recordings of children or parent-child interactions,[46] or to quickly search a child's electronic medical record for information that could assign a higher prior probability for interpreting the screening results.[47] These "Artificial Intelligence" assisted approaches would be limited by the diversity within the data from which they learned, but perhaps over time could achieve better degrees of sensitivity and specificity than current brief screeners.

From the point of view of treatability; however, one major limitation of current screening is that by focusing on "diagnostic" levels of symptoms it turns attention away from issues that are either already causing functional difficulty or that are likely to do so if left unattended.[48] For example, a study of 4 to 9 year olds in Connecticut primary care practices found that 14% of children assessed had "subthreshold" diagnoses (that is, they would have been missed by the standard screen had their parents not been asked separately about functioning); 20% of these children progressed to having a "full" disorder a year later.[49]

Current screening is also problematic in that it tries to identify particular conditions that are thought to have specific treatments. This is consistent with both medical models that match treatment to condition and with the emphasis on evidence-based care within mental health (where most evidence comes from studies of particular populations with rigorously-defined diagnoses). However, as they emerge, mental health problems in children take on many forms that often poorly predict future illness states. For example, irritability in young children and anhedonia in youth are symptoms that non-specifically predict later functional problems and disorders, and most importantly, could be targets of early intervention.[50–53]

Another difficulty with processes related to screening—stepped-care and 'treatment to target" which are foundations of collaborative primary care approaches to mental health, but also with important ethical stances of first using least restrictive or least risky treatments—is that it can take time to match the correct range and intensity of treatment to a patient or family's needs. This is a special problem in primary care where there is very limited time to explore a full range of symptoms, strengths, and vulnerabilities at the time problems initially present. Screening for social determinants of health, adverse childhood events, and parental mental health problems may partly address this dilemma, but work is in process to develop methods for better understanding the extent of intervention required—whether it would be considered prevention or treatment. Enhanced screening tools (likely digital) might be deployed in primary care and help determine if patients should rapidly be referred on to specialty care or brief interventions in collaborative care rather than having to "fail" earlier steps.[54,55]

CONSENSUS THAT PSYCHOLOGIC THERAPIES NEED TO BE MADE MORE EFFECTIVE

Over the last few years, the Wellcome Trust in the UK commissioned a worldwide effort to identify "active ingredients" in the psychologic treatments that are commonly used to help children and youth.[56,57] A major goal was to find interventions that might be readily deployed across settings serving young people—including primary care. Wellcome explored a wide-range of interventions that they lumped into 6 groups, some of which map closely on to the ingredients of evidence-based psychotherapies and others that were more related to social determinants of health. Their overall conclusion was that while many of the interventions had good evidence supporting their effectiveness, overall effectiveness was modest and that there were no clear "front runners" with large effects or that appeared to be universally applicable. They concluded that different combinations off these "ingredients" would likely be needed for different individuals in different communities.

The Wellcome conclusions fit with the observation that current understandings of the cognitive processes that underlie mood and behavior problems are not yet specific enough to develop stronger treatments. For example, Pile and colleagues[58] developed an intervention for adolescent depression based on the association of negative and positive mental autobiographic memories with depression onset and persistence. Another project is attempting to understand which brain areas are involved and which mental processes are altered when anxious children and adolescents respond (or do not) to cognitive behavioral therapy.[59]

The uncertainty about mechanisms of action and ability to predict who will respond extends to medications.[60] US and UK recommendations vary on the necessity of pairing medication treatment with therapy, in part because of differences in access to therapy in between the 2 health care systems. Some work in neuroscience suggests that selective serotonin reuptake inhibitors do not work independently of psychosocial mechanisms—they change the way we perceive cues in the environment ("affective bias")—and so they are best paired with psychosocial interventions, or their effectiveness can be to some extent predicted by psychosocial context.[61]

ORGANIZING PRINCIPLES FOR A FUTURE PEDIATRIC MENTAL HEALTH SYSTEM

The future pediatric mental health system will be the product of systematic, deliberate planning at local and state/province/regional levels. Governments will find that it "pays" to do this systematically in terms of building responsive systems and generating the political will to sustain them.[62] In British Columbia, a province-wide initiative funded centrally but carried out by local collaboratives—centered on families and youth—was able to find local solutions to big problems in the pediatric mental health care system.[63] Relationships at the local level were a key, with new structures emerging from small changes among many different clinical and community stakeholders. But it took effort to keep the work focused on mutual wins and to maintain the urgency of coming up with something new.

Systems of the future will build communities that support child, youth, and family mental health through their structure and institutions. This is not a new idea, but it is one that needs constant nurturing. The built environment facilitates social interaction, recreation, and healing green spaces.[64] Policies promote affordable housing and locally-owned small business, which promotes stable neighborhoods with high social capital,[65,66] and there are publicly-supported facilities that provide young people and families with opportunities for recreation and socializing. The clinical community has a presence at many of these facilities, just as it now has a presence in many Head Start Centers and schools. Expansion of early child care and pre-school programs have long been seen as foundations of child mental health,[67] as well as restoration of schools as hubs for a range of universally accessible educational and recreational activities that help to develop skills, recognize multiple intelligences, and social connectedness.[68] For adolescents, models like SODO in Japan illustrate how community centers can become gateways to mental health services and sites where young people can in formal and informal ways connect with supportive peers.[69]

In the future, primary care, rather than community mental health facilities, will be seen as the home of clinical mental health programs for children and youth. This shift will occur because of the recognition that prevention and early treatment are essential to reducing the burden of mental health problems and helping families flourish, and that primary care is the place where near-universal access, longitudinal care, and a truly integrating focus all converge. Several things will have to have to fall into place to make this shift happen.

First, primary care clinicians will need to have more confidence in their own ability to promote mental health and to detect and treat emerging problems. Currently practicing clinicians will gain this confidence through ongoing support via integrated care and on-demand informal consultation mechanisms that will either be built into integrated care or available at a regional or state level.[70] Advances in computerized assessment of conversations will make it possible for them to train more easily and/or to submit recorded clips from actual visits (with consent) to learn new skills or polish existing one.[71] The rising generations of primary care clinicians will learn more mental health skills as a part of their residency training, though if these skills are to be oriented toward early intervention and treatment, residency programs will, as in other specialties, need to find time to provide the training in continuity and outpatient settings rather than providing it only in the context of emergency and inpatient services.[72] In addition, even physicians working in medical subspecialities will believe that addressing the mental health of their patients—especially those with serious, chronic conditions—should be part of their competencies.[73]

To support primary care as a core mental health function, the concept of integrated care will be enlarged to encompass functions that are now usually implemented separately. Every primary care practice will be a base for a range of clinicians who can provide first-line care for parental mood and substance problems,[74] link families to resources required to meet basic needs, support early childhood relationships (especially for families whose children have emerging developmental challenges), and provide first-line treatment for emerging emotional and behavioral problems in older children.[75] The need for these types of care is sufficiently prevalent in primary care that the barriers posed by providing them through referral cannot be justified.

These primary care-based clinicians will need to have the right tools at their disposal.[48] This will include new tools for screening and new models of initial treatment that are not tied to diagnoses but rather to both the underlying cognitive and social drivers of individual's problems and to the chief functional problems families face. Primary care clinicians and their teams will be experts in coaching families to use self-help materials that are tailored to their needs.[20] Screening for strengths and vulnerabilities in social development will be central part of early assessments and will be linked to support for parenting and to suggestions for early childhood care providers and educators.[76] Primary care will also need new tools to rapidly assess for cognitive problems that interfere with learning in school,[77] and it will need staff members particularly tasked and skilled in working with school systems. It will also need practical but sophisticated information systems that, with the collaboration of families, will allow for the creation of registries and mechanisms for monitoring both wellness and the status of identified problems.

There is reason to believe that these primary care sites will need to be relatively small and anchored in the communities that they serve. Teams need to know each other, share overlapping functions, and be capable of flexing in real time.[34] Truly integrated systems rely on human-to-human interactions.[78] Practices need to know their communities and be seen as knowing by the community. That knowing includes having a population-based mission and staff that makes the facility a visible presence outside the facility doors. There is a strong "back to the future" component to this vision. It is the model on which effective systems in other countries have been based (for example, Brazil's Family Health Strategy)[79] and the community health center movement in the US.[80] A group in Massachusetts has in recent years taken on the specific task of bringing integrated pediatric mental health care into community health centers.[81]

It may take time (and seeing what parallel reforms happen for the adult mental health system) to understand if these community-based primary care practices should retain their focus on families with children versus looking more like health centers that provide care across the lifespan. As the population ages, life-span oriented centers will face even greater challenges than they do today providing close attention to the needs of families living with chronic health and cognitive conditions at later stages of life, which historically has been in competition for resources with care for families with young children.

In the future, some (or maybe most) communities will need to evolve another layer of mental health support that sits between primary care and the very specialized mental health services that target individuals with significant chronic disability or more well-defined conditions amenable to specific treatments (for example, intensive treatment for obsessive-compulsive disorder, or dialectical behavioral therapy for persistent self-harm). This layer is emerging in some vertically integrated systems in the US[82] and is a component of pilot community-based systems in the Netherlands.[36] Some of the larger state "access programs" includes components such as the ability to refer a patient for a 1-time psychiatric assessment.[70] But in addition to assessment, the added layer provides a venue for transdiagnostic treatment designed to either enable a family to return to primary care or move efficiently into a higher level of service (**Table 2**). The middle layer has to operate with a high degree of trust from clinicians above and below it. At the primary care level, clinicians have to feel confident that families returned to them can be safely cared for, and that the middle layer clinicians will

Table 2
Limits to screening, diagnosis, and treatment; future responses

Forces Driving Change	Responses of a Future System
Problems with current screening	
• Low predictive value • Cut-offs identify those already having considerable impact • Overly focused on specific conditions when most child problems span current diagnostic categories • Don't help identify individuals not likely to respond to first line treatments (likely to "fail" first parts of stepped care)	• New screening tools target both capacities that underly successful development (for example social development) and transdiagnostic symptoms (irritability, anhedonia) • Tools that better target transdiagnostic issues of primary concern to patients and families • New tools that identify both current symptom level and help stratify youth or families into levels of need for first-line treatment
Problems with current therapies	
• Small effect sizes • Treatment often too late—misses windows when prevention likely • Lack of relatively universal interventions; need tailoring • High proportion of "treatment resistant" individuals for psychotherapy and psychopharmacology • Lack of integration of mental health interventions with substance treatment or treatment of developmental and cognitive problems	• More deliberate training in and on-going support for clinicians' use of 'common factors' associated with outcomes across treatment modalities • Treatment plans that include attention to social determinants and problems of other family members that interact with the patient's problems • Coached self-help interventions as practical ways to tailor treatment and increase intensity • Enhanced methods for monitoring and preventing relapse • New treatments based on better understanding of underlying mechanisms (such as pairing interventions that promote plasticity with psychotherapies) • Tertiary systems focus less on crises (which are better served in community settings) and more on acute/severe illness and treatment-resistance
Primary care workforce issues	
• Lack of confidence in mental health skills • Lack of integration with mental health care system	• Basing expanded, multi-generational mental health team in primary care; expanded integrated care model • Increased inclusion on teams of peers and community health workers who can deliver or coach treatments in multiple languages and cultural frames • Mental health training for medical generalists focused on early detection and treatment • Organizing community mental health system as 'hub' for primary care practices

be an ongoing source of support. At the specialist level, clinicians have to trust the middle layer to make appropriate diagnoses and know which form of specialty care is required. The payoff for primary and specialty care is efficiency. Primary care practices have a single point of referral for families that are out of their scope; specialty clinicians do not need to take time for extensive evaluations prior to starting treatment.

The "middle layer" model may be best where it could grow naturally by redefining the roles and treatment modalities of community mental health centers, and where there are tertiary facilities (for example, children's hospitals with mental health programs) that provide very specialized services. In these communities, rather than trying to provide a range of evidence-based specific interventions, community mental health sites would focus on transdiagnostic treatments (with additional resources for further addressing social determinants and educational issues), and leave more specific care for tertiary centers. In smaller communities with less access to specialty services, the model may rely more on community mental health centers as providing both transdiagnostic and specialty care. For example, in Iran, community mental health centers anchor networks of general practitioner (GP) offices within a catchment area, providing the GPs with training and supervision in brief mental health care, supporting registries, and facilitating treatment at the centers when needed.[83]

Tertiary mental health care will also change. Most importantly, it will address the fact that its most successful treatments in many cases continue to yield only partial improvements or fail to significantly help large proportions of those coming for care.[60] Tertiary mental health programs struggle with the same problems as lower levels of care trying to balance the need for long-term support of individuals and families with promoting treatment and "discharge" to open room for the newly referred. Barring major advances in treatment, tertiary systems (and state payers) of the near future will need to develop programs that provide long-term support for families with complex problems. Community-based "wrap around" services are available in some areas, but they have shown positive but limited effectiveness in terms of impact on mental health symptoms and functioning.[84] Enhanced models may be needed that can provide care for longer periods of time and that coordinate more closely with treating clinicians at the tertiary site. Tertiary sites will also need to develop the kinds of research networks and infrastructure that characterize pediatric oncology, for example, so that trials of novel interventions such as those pairing neural plasticity with psychologic interventions can be rapidly developed and made accessible.[85]

HOW CAN CHANGE HAPPEN?

A product of the way many health care systems are financed and grow is that resources appear in places that clinicians want to live and where communities have a tax and income base to support them. Though again not a new idea, planning still does not consistently involve processes for modeling where to best place (or support existing) services to serve particular communities,[86] and now, with the growth of telehealth, how to balance the use of in-person and tele services to optimize services and resources.[87] Targeted support for sites in areas of greatest need can also address one of the greatest implementation challenges for integrated care and similar services, which is that sites that experience the most stress from underfinancing or high patient acuity are often those that have the least capacity to undertake change, and are less likely to participate in practice transformation opportunities.[88]

Support for those making changes to community-based practices will need to include solid financing. Practices need financial assistance at start-up of new services,[89] and some costs related to providing fully integrated care may need ongoing subsidies under the current financing systems.[90] Some of this ongoing cost could be saved with implementation support that goes beyond current learning collaborative models,[91] which can be effective but also take considerable participant time,[92] and risk not sufficiently engaging community and consumer voices. It may also take more resolve at a federal level. In the US, attempts at system reform such as the InCK program or the CCMHC model for community mental health tend to be implemented in ways that make them optional for the individual states. In contrast, the nationwide CYPIAPT program in the UK was able to make substantial and relatively uniform improvements to the organization and implementation of child and youth mental health services.[93]

The future will also include health services experiments that challenge potentially false beliefs about how to deliver mental health care in a cost-effective manner. Trials will test whether clinics—especially those serving disadvantaged populations – can better implement evidence-based practices if they receive sufficient funding.[94] Other trials will test the proposition that the most efficient care (that is, that achieves the best outcomes for the most people) may not be the highest possible volume but rather care at a pace that optimizes client-clinician relationships and allows time for clinicians to participate in supervision and other quality-enhancing activities that take time but improve outcomes.[95]

SUMMARY

An optimistic view of the future child/youth mental health system is that it will be shaped in part by innovations in early detection and treatment of functional problems, coupled with the power of digital technology to provide new ways to help individuals and families monitor their well-being and seek or agree to help as it is needed. These innovations; however, will be deployed within a community-based health care system that fully implements ideas that have been around for decades and that over time, have been partially implemented but then periodically challenged, usually by forces linked to the business of medicine or by shifting political views on the scope of government's role in promoting social welfare. What might finally overcome these challenges is the sense that the ground is literally shifting underneath our feet. In countries across the world, and in states within the US, populations are rapidly changing in their age and ethnic composition. Climate change, regardless of one's view of its origins, is generating a sense among younger generations that the status quo is untenable.[96] It is also possible that governments will push back against the extreme concentration of wealth that has had a role in the health problems that stem from inequality and partially transferred control of health policy to donors with sufficient resources that they can influence the direction even of major international health care agencies.[97] As in the past, it will likely be the pairing of the properly-articulated case with the right grass-roots advocacy and highly-placed political skills that will make the paradigm-shifting change possible.[98]

CLINICS CARE POINTS

- Growing the mental health capacity of primary care continues to offer the most promising path to increasing access to child/youth mental health services.
- Relying on diagnostic thresholds, as is the practice in current screening proceesses, may fail to identify children/youth who are already experiencing considerable problems with functioning.

- The social determinants of health are major drivers of current and future mental health status and need to be parts of every differential diagnosis and treatment plan.
- It is difficult or impossible to address a child's mental health problem without an appreciation of and providing support for the mental health and social challenges of their caregivers; purely pediatric practices need to find ways of addressing caregivers' mental health needs.
- At this point in time, only primary care provides the long-term follow-up required for the care of most child/youth mental health problems, as well as the holistic somatic, developmental, and social care required for adequate mental health treatment.

DISCLOSURE

The authors have nothing to disclose.

FUNDING

Dr Wissow's work on this paper was partially supported by an anonymous gift to the Seattle Children's Hospital Foundation in support of evaluating new models for delivering early community-based child and youth mental health services.

REFERENCES

1. Strauss V. The greatest commencement speech ever. The Washington Post 2014.
2. Kohrt BA, Ottman K, Panter-Brick C, et al. Why we heal: The evolution of psychological healing and implications for global mental health. Clin Psychol Rev 2020;82:101920.
3. Natarajan A, Moslimani M, Lopez MH. Key facts about recent trends in global migration. Pew Research Center, 2022. Available at: https://www.pewresearch.org/short-reads/2022/12/16/key-facts-about-recent-trends-in-global-migration/. Accessed March 15, 2024.
4. Available at: https://data.unicef.org/topic/child-migration-and-displacement/displacement/. Accessed March 15, 2024.
5. Barghadouch A, Carlsson J, Norredam M. Psychiatric disorders and predictors hereof among refugee children in early adulthood: A register-based cohort study. J Nerv Ment Dis 2018;206:3–10.
6. Available at: https://www.stlouisfed.org/open-vault/2024/feb/us-wealth-inequality-widespread-gains-gaps-remain. Accessed March 15, 2024.
7. Dickman SL, Himmelstein DU, Woolhandler S. Inequality and the health-care system in the USA. Lancet 2017;389:1431–41.
8. Reiss F, Meyrose AK, Otto C, et al. Socioeconomic status, stressful life situations and mental health problems in children and adolescents: Results of the German BELLA cohort-study. PLoS One 2019;14:e0213700.
9. Marmot M, Goldblatt P, Allen J, et al. Fair Society, health lives. The Marmot review. Strategic review of health inequalities in england post-2010. London: University College London; 2010.
10. Ford K, von Russdorf S, Ahlborn L. Unlocking potential: how social protection can improve disadvantaged children's foundational cognitive skills. Policy Brief 59. Oxford: Young Lives, 2023.
11. Ford K, von Russdorf S. Weathering the storm: climate shocks threaten children's skills and learning but social programs can mitigate impact. Young Lives Policy Brief 61. Oxford: Oxford Department of International Development; 2023.

12. Pazos N, Favara M, Sánchez A, et al. Long-term effects of rainfall shocks on foundational cognitive skills: evidence from Peru, PIER working paper 23-001. Philadelphia: Penn Institute for Economic Researc; 2023. Available at: https://economics.sas.upenn.edu/system/files/working-papers/23-001%20PIER%20Paper%20.Submission.pdf. Accessed November 28, 2023.
13. Chang G, Favara M, Novella R. The origins of cognitive skills and personality: the effect of in-utero climate shocks on adolescents and young adult life outcomes. Econ Hum Biol 2022;44:101089.
14. Rossiter J, Woodhead M, Rolleston C, et al. Delivering on every child's right to basic skills (Executive Summary). Oxford: Young Lives; 2018.
15. UNESCO. The right to education in the 21st Century. Findings from the International Seminar on the Evolving Right to Education. December 7-8, 2021. Available at: https://unesdoc.unesco.org/ark:/48223/pf0000381108/PDF/381108eng.pdf.multi. Accessed April 1, 2024.
16. UNESCO Insititute for Statistics. More than one-half of children and adolescents are not learning worldwide. Fact sheet 46. Montreal: UNESCO Institute for Statistics; 2017.
17. US Department of Education 2023 Equity Action Plan Summary (February, 2023).
18. Williams JC, Ball M, Roscoe N, et al. Widening racial disparities during COVID-19 telemedicine transition: a study of child mental health services at two large children's hospitals. J Am Acad Child Adolesc Psychiatry 2023;62:447–56.
19. Kuroda N, Burkey MD, Wissow LS. Discovering common elements of empirically supported self-help interventions for depression in primary care: a systematic review. J Gen Intern Med 2021;36:869–80.
20. van Doorn M, Nijhuis LA, Egeler MD, et al. Online indicated preventive mental health interventions for youth: a scoping review. Front Psychiatry 2021;12:580843.
21. van Doorn M, Nijhuis LA, Monsanto A, et al. Usability, feasibility, and effect of a biocueing intervention in addition to a moderated digital social therapy-platform in young people with emerging mental health problems: a mixed-method approach. Front Psychiatry 2022;13:871813.
22. Cross SP, Scott JL, Hermens DF, et al. Variability in clinical outcomes for youths treated for subthreshold severe mental disorders at an Early Intervention Service. Psychiatr Serv 2018;69:555–61.
23. Hickie IB, Davenport TA, Burns JM, et al. Project Synergy: co-designing technology-enabled solutions for Australian mental health services reform. Med J Aust 2019;211(Suppl 7):S3–39.
24. Lasswell, Sophie. Financial Inaccessibility of Mental Healthcare in the United States. Ballard Brief. 2022. Available at: www.ballardbrief.byu.edu. Accessed April 1, 2024.
25. Stewart RE, Adams DR, Mandell DS, et al. The perfect storm: collision of the business of mental health and the implementation of evidence-based practices. Psychiatr Serv 2016;67:159–61.
26. Beidas RS, Marcus S, Wolk CB, et al. A prospective examination of clinician and supervisor turnover within the context of implementation of evidence-based practices in a publicly-funded mental health system. Adm Policy Ment Health 2016;43:640–9.
27. Available at: https://www.who.int/news-room/fact-sheets/detail/universal-health-coverage-(uhc). Accessed April 1, 2024.
28. Schleider JL, Dobias ML, Sung JY, et al. Future directions in single- session youth mental health interventions. J Clin Child Adolesc Psychol 2020;49:264–78.

29. Bauer AM, Thielke SM, Katon W, et al. Aligning health information technologies with effective service delivery models to improve chronic disease care. Prev Med 2014;66:167–72.
30. Beaulieu ND, Dafny LS, Landon BE, et al. Changes in quality of care after hospital mergers and acquisitions. N Engl J Med 2020;382:51–9.
31. Bravo F, Braun M, Farias V, et al. Optimization-driven framework to understand health care network costs and resource allocation. Health Care Manag Sci 2021;24:640–60.
32. Bunger AC, Choi MS, MacDowell H, et al. Competition among mental health organizations: environmental drivers and strategic responses. Adm Policy Ment Health 2021;48:393–407.
33. Dambi JM, Mavhu W, Beji-Chauke R, et al. The impact of working alliance in managing youth anxiety and depression: a scoping review. Npj Ment Health Res. 2023;2:1.
34. Leykum LK, Lanham HJ, Pugh JA, et al. Manifestations and implications of uncertainty for improving healthcare systems: an analysis of observational and interventional studies grounded in complexity science. Implement Sci 2014;9:165.
35. Kirkbride JB, Anglin DM, Colman I, et al. The social determinants of mental health and disorder: evidence, prevention and recommendations. World Psychiatr 2024; 23:58–90.
36. Available at: https://www.nji.nl/sites/default/files/2021-06/Reform-of-the-Dutch-system-for-child-and-youth-care.pdf. Accessed April 1, 2024.
37. Shared Intelligence. Action to address health inequalities in Greater London and the Mayoral combined authorities. 2020. Available at: https://www.health.org.uk/sites/default/files/2022-06/action_to_address_health_inequalities_in_greater_london_and_the_mayoral_combined_authorities.pdf. Accessed April 30, 2024.
38. Vanneste YTM, Lanting CI, Detmar SB. The preventive child and youth healthcare service in the Netherlands: The state of the art and challenges ahead. Int J Environ Res Public Health 2022;19:8736.
39. Jones EB, Lucienne TM. The Integrated Care for Kids model: addressing fragmented care for pediatric Medicaid enrollees in seven communities. J Health Care Poor Underserved 2023;34:503–9.
40. James G, Kasper E, Wong CA, et al. Investing in child health through alternative payment models: lessons from North Carolina Integrated Care for Kids. Med Care Res Rev 2023;29. 10775587231217178.
41. Cuijpers P, Weitz E, Karyotaki E, et al. The effects of psychological treatment of maternal depression on children and parental functioning: a meta-analysis. Eur Child Adolesc Psychiatry 2015;24:237–45.
42. Furlong M, McGilloway S, Bywater T, et al. Behavioural and cognitive-behavioural group- based parenting programmes for early-onset conduct problems in children aged 3 to 12 years. Cochrane Database Syst Rev 2012;(2). Art. No.: CD008225.
43. Lipari RN, Van Horn SL. Children living with parents who have a substance use disorder. The CBHSQ Report. Rockville, MD: SAMSHA; 2017.
44. Velleman R, Templeton LJ. Impact of parents' substance misuse on children: an update. BJPsych Adv 2016;22:108–17.
45. Lavigne JV, Feldman M, Meyers KM. Screening for mental health problems: addressing the base rate fallacy for a sustainable screening program in integrated primary care. J Pediatr Psychol 2016;41:1081–90.
46. Abbas H, Garberson F, Liu-Mayo S, et al. Multi-modular AI approach to streamline autism diagnosis in young children. Sci Rep 2020;10:5014.

47. Cortez AB, Wilkins J, Handler E, et al. Multistage adolescent depression screening: a comparison of 11-year-olds to 12-year-olds. Perm J 2021; 25(20):233.
48. Colizzi M, Lasalvia A, Ruggeri M. Prevention and early intervention in youth mental health: is it time for a multidisciplinary and trans-diagnostic model for care? Int J Ment Health Syst 2020;14:23.
49. Briggs-Gowan MJ, Owens PL, Schwab-Stone ME, et al. Persistence of psychiatric disorders in pediatric settings. J Am Acad Child Adolesc Psychiatry 2003;42: 1360–9.
50. Wiggins JL, Ureña Rosario A, Zhang Y, et al. Advancing earlier transdiagnostic identification of mental health risk: A pragmatic approach at the transition to toddlerhood. Int J Methods Psychiatr Res 2023;32(S1):e1989.
51. Freed RD, Mehra LM, Laor D, et al. Anhedonia as a clinical correlate of inflammation in adolescents across psychiatric conditions. World J Biol Psychiatry 2019; 20:712–22.
52. Pizzagalli DA. Depression, stress, and anhedonia: toward a synthesis and integrated model. Annu Rev Clin Psychol 2014;10:393–423.
53. McGorry PD, Hartmann JA, Spooner R, et al. Beyond the "at risk mental state" concept: transitioning to transdiagnostic psychiatry. World Psychiatr 2018;17: 133–42.
54. Shah JL, Scott J, McGorry PD, et al. Transdiagnostic clinical staging in youth mental health: a first international consensus statement. World Psychiatr 2020; 19:233–42.
55. Chong MK, Hickie IB, Cross SP, et al. Digital application of clinical staging to support stratification in youth mental health services: validity and reliability study. JMIR Form Res 2023;7:e45161.
56. Wellcome Trust. What science has shown can help young people with anxiety and depression. Identifying and reviewing the 'active ingredients' of effective interventions: Part 1, 2021. Zenodo. Available at: https://doi.org/10.5281/zenodo.7327137. Accessed April 30, 2024.
57. Wellcome. Trust. What science has shown can help young people with anxiety and depression. Identifying and reviewing the 'active ingredients' of effective interventions: Part 2, 2022. Zenodo. Available at: https://doi.org/10.5281/zenodo.7327296. Accessed April 30, 2024.
58. Pile V, Smith P, Leamy M, et al. A feasibility randomised controlled trial of a brief early intervention for adolescent depression that targets emotional mental images and memory specificity (IMAGINE). Behav Res Ther 2021;143:103876.
59. Premo JE, Liu Y, Bilek EL, et al. Grant report on anxiety-CBT: dimensional brain behavior predictors of CBT outcomes in pediatric anxiety. J Psychiatry Brain Sci 2020;5:e200005. Available at: https://jpbs.hapres.com/htmls/JPBS_1195_Detail.html#sec9. Accessed April 30, 2024.
60. Dwyer JB, Stringaris A, Brent DA, et al. Annual research review: defining and treating pediatric treatment-resistant depression. J Child Psychol Psychiatry 2020;61:312–32.
61. Murphy SE, Capitão LP, Giles SLC, et al. The knowns and unknowns of SSRI treatment in young people with depression and anxiety: efficacy, predictors, and mechanisms of action. Lancet Psychiatr 2021;8:824–35.
62. Halsall T, Manion I, Mathias S, et al. Frayme: Building the structure to support the international spread of integrated youth services. Early Interv Psychiatry 2020;14: 495–502.

63. Mullens A, Nehra L. Legacy: progress of the Child and Youth Mental Health and Substance Abuse Collaborative. Doctors of BC and the British Columbia Government. 2017. Available at: https://collaborativetoolbox.ca/legacy-magazine. Accessed April 30, 2024.
64. Healthy Liverpool, the Blueprint. Liverpool clinical commissioning group. Liverpool; 2015.
65. Sampson RJ, Raudenbush SW, Earls F. Neighborhoods and violent crime: a multilevel study of collective efficacy. Science 1997;277:918–24.
66. Fuller T. Public Housing Helps Paris Stay Paris. N Y Times 2024. Section RE, Page 9.
67. Shonkoff JP, Boyce WT, Levitt P, et al. Leveraging the biology of adversity and resilience to transform pediatric practice. Pediatrics 2021;147:e20193845.
68. Cohen J, McCabe L, Michelli NM, et al. School climate: Research, policy, practice, and teacher education. Teach Coll Rec 2009;111:180–213.
69. Uchino T, Kotsuji Y, Kitano T, et al. An integrated youth mental health service in a densely populated metropolitan area in Japan: clinical case management bridges the gap between mental health and illness services. Early Interv Psychiatry 2022;16:568–75.
70. Mazur SL, Edelsohn GA, DePergola PA 2nd, et al. Ethical imperatives for participation in integrated/collaborative care models for pediatric mental health care. Child Adolesc Psychiatr Clin N Am 2021;30:697–712.
71. Creed TA, Salama L, Slevin R, et al. Enhancing the quality of cognitive behavioral therapy in community mental health through artificial intelligence generated fidelity feedback (Project AFFECT): a study protocol. BMC Health Serv Res 2022;22:1177.
72. St. Geme JW. Proposed 2024 pediatrics requirements, April 5, 2023. Available at: https://media.amspdc.org/wp-content/uploads/2023/05/10154414/2024-Pediatric-Requirements-AMSPDC-Response.pdf. Accessed April 30, 2024.
73. Green C, Leyenaar JK, Leslie LK. Association between educational resources and pediatric fellows' mental health attitudes and self-reported competence. Acad Pediatr 2023;23:1628–35.
74. Bosk EA, Van Scoyoc A, Mihalec-Adkins B, et al. Integrating responses to caregiver substance misuse, intimate partner violence and child maltreatment: Initiatives and policies that support families at risk for entering the child welfare system. Aggress Violent Behav 2022;65:101637.
75. Renn BN, Casey C, Raue PJ, et al. Task sharing to expand access to care: development of a behavioral health support specialist. Psychiatr Serv 2023;74:76–8.
76. Willis DW, Condon MC, Moe V, et al. The context and development of the early relational health screen. Infant Ment Health J 2022;43:493–506.
77. Willcutt EG, Boada R, Riddle MW, et al. Colorado Learning Difficulties Questionnaire: Validation of a parent-report screening measure. Psychological Assessmen 2011;23:778–91.
78. Brown JD, King MA, Wissow LS. The central role of relationships with trauma-informed integrated care for children and youth. Acad Pediatr 2017;17(7S): S94–101.
79. Macinko J, Mendonça CS. Estratégia Saúde da Família, um forte modelo de Atenção Primária à Saúde que traz resultados.[The family health strategy, a powerful model for primary health care that brings results]. Saúde Debate 2018;42(special number):18–37.
80. Rosenbaum S, Tolbert J, Sharac J, et al. Community health centers: growing importance in a changing health care system. Washington, DC: Kaiser Family Foundation; 2018.

81. Kim J, Sheldrick RC, Gallagher K, et al. Association of integrating mental health into pediatric primary care at Federally Qualified Health Centers with utilization and follow-up care. JAMA Netw Open 2023;6:e239990.
82. Schweitzer J, Bird A, Bowers H, et al. Developing an innovative pediatric integrated mental health care program: interdisciplinary team successes and challenges. Front Psychiatry 2023;14:1252037.
83. Sharifi V, Shahrivar Z, Zarafshan H, et al. Effect of general practitioner training in a collaborative child mental health care program on children's mental health outcomes in a low-resource setting: a cluster randomized trial. JAMA Psychiatr 2023;80:22–30.
84. Olson JR, Benjamin PH, Azman AA, et al. Systematic review and meta-analysis: effectiveness of wraparound care coordination for children and adolescents. J Am Acad Child Adolesc Psychiatry 2021;60:1353–66.
85. McEwen BS, Akil H. Revisiting the stress concept: implications for affective disorders. J Neurosci 2020;40:12–21.
86. Griffin PM, Scherrer CR, Want JL. Optimization of community health center locations and service offerings with statistical need estimation. ILE transactions 2008; 40:880–92.
87. Musdal H, Shiner B, Chen T, et al. In-person and video-based post-traumatic stress disorder treatment for veterans: a location-allocation model. Mil Med 2014;179:150–6.
88. King MA, Wissow LS, Baum RA. The role of organizational context in the implementation of a statewide initiative to integrate mental health services into pediatric primary care. Health Care Manag Rev 2018;43:206–17.
89. Meadows Mental Health Policy Institute. Improving Behavioral Health Care for Youth Through Collaborative Care Expansion. Final Report. 2023.
90. Walter HJ, Vernacchio L, Trudell EK, et al. Five-year outcomes of behavioral health integration in pediatric primary care. Pediatrics 2019;144:e20183243.
91. Schleider JL, Beidas RS. Harnessing the single-session intervention approach to promote scalable implementation of evidence-based practices in healthcare. Front Health Serv 2022;2:997406.
92. Gotham HJ, Paris M Jr, Hoge MA. Learning collaboratives: a strategy for quality improvement and implementation in behavioral health. J Behav Health Serv Res 2023;50:263–78.
93. Ludlow C, Hurn R, Lansdell S. A current review of the Children and Young People's Improving Access to Psychological Therapies (CYP IAPT) program: perspectives on developing an accessible workforce. Adolesc Health Med Ther 2020;11:21–8.
94. Stewart RE, Mandell DS, Beidas RS. Lessons from Maslow: prioritizing funding to improve the quality of community mental health and substance use services. Psychiatr Serv 2021;72:1219–21.
95. Schriger SH, Becker-Haimes EM, Skriner L, et al. Clinical supervision in community mental health: characterizing supervision as usual and exploring predictors of supervision content and process. Community Ment Health J 2021;57:552–66.
96. Schwartz SEO, Benoit L, Clayton S, et al. Climate change anxiety and mental health: environmental activism as buffer. Curr Psychol 2022;28:1–14.
97. Kerdellant C. Ces milliardaires plus forts que les états. [These billionaires more powerful than countries]. Paris: Editions-Observatoire; 2024.
98. Redman E. The dance of legislation. New York: Simon and Schuster; 1973.